Sexually Transmitted Diseases

Derek Llewellyn-Jones is an acknowledged expert in the field of sexual medicine. He is the author of many successful books for the general reader and for the medical profession. Among his best known books are *Everywoman*, *Breastfeeding: How to Succeed*, and *Fundamentals of Obstetrics and Gynaecology*. He was until recently Associate Professor of Obstetrics and Gynaecology at the University of Sydney.

By the same author

EVERYWOMAN

BREASTFEEDING: HOW TO SUCCEED

FUNDAMENTALS OF OBSTETRICS AND GYNAECOLOGY
Vol. 1 OBSTETRICS
Vol. 2 GYNAECOLOGY

Sexually Transmitted Diseases

Derek Llewellyn-Jones OBE, MD, MAO, FRCOG, FRACOG

faber and faber
LONDON · BOSTON

First published in 1985
as *Herpes, Aids and Other Sexually Transmitted Diseases*
This revised edition published in 1990
by Faber and Faber Limited
3 Queen Square, London WC1N 3AU

Photoset by Wilmaset Birkenhead Wirral
Printed in Great Britain
by Clays Ltd, St Ives plc

A CIP record of this book
is available from the British Library

ISBN 0-571-14418-7

To the memory of Philippe Ricord, born in 1799, and died in 1889, an eminent venereologist who finally identified that gonorrhoea and syphilis were two separate diseases, and of whom Oliver Wendell Holmes wrote 'he was the Voltaire of pelvic literature – a skeptic as to the mortality of the race in general, who would have submitted Diana to treatment with his specifics and ordered a course of blue pills for the Vestal Virgins'.

VD is not primarily a medical problem. It is instead a social one dependent on those factors which most influence attitudes and behaviour.

G. Hart, *Sexual Maladjustment and Disease*
(Chicago: Nelson Hall, 1977)

Contents

Illustrations and Tables

ILLUSTRATIONS

TABLES

Glossary

ABORTION The expulsion from the uterus of the fetus before the end of the 20th week of pregnancy. The expulsion may occur spontaneously (when the process is often called a 'miscarriage'), or be induced by a doctor.

AFTERBIRTH The placenta.

ANAEROBIC Not needing oxygen for growth and survival.

'CARRIER' A person who has no symptoms of an infectious disease but may, in certain circumstances, infect another.

CERVICAL CANCER Cancer of the neck of the uterus; the most common gynaecological cancer in women.

CHANCRE A small ulcer usually found on the outer genitals. A 'hard' chancre (which has a raised firm edge surrounding the ulcer) is due to syphilis.

CHLAMYDIA A virus-like organism.

COITUS Sexual intercourse.

CONTACT-TRACING The process of seeking sexual contacts of people infected with syphilis or gonorrhoea so that they may be checked to find whether they are also infected.

COPULATION Making love, having sex.

DOUCHE A procedure of washing out the vagina for 'hygienic' purposes. Previously fashionable in the USA, it is not much used today as it has no real value.

GANGLION A bean-shaped area in a nerve near the spinal cord, where the nerve fibres relay.

HIV (Human Immunodeficiency Virus) The virus responsible for AIDS.

IMMUNE SYSTEM The system of cells and circulating substances (antibodies) which protects the body against invasion by 'foreign' proteins in the form of viruses, bacteria or, occasionally, food substances.

LYMPH NODES 'Staging areas' in the lymphatic system where infective agents are often held up. This leads to swelling of the node. Also called 'lymph glands'.

MISCARRIAGE See abortion.

OPPORTUNISTIC INFECTIONS Infections that are usually easily controlled, but, if the immune defences of the body are weak, grow rapidly or 'opportunistically'.

ORGASM The climax of a sexual encounter.

PAP SMEAR A swab taken from the cervix of the uterus to detect abnormal cells which may indicate an early cancer.

PLACEBO An innocuous substance given to 'humour' a patient, or for psychological reasons when no effective treatment is available. Also used as a 'control' in trials of new drugs. Placebos relieve symptoms in many cases, particularly of psychosomatic illness.

SEXUALITY The sum of a person's inherited make-up: knowledge, experiences, attitudes and behaviours as they relate to being a woman or a man. It includes those ways of behaving that increase love between two people.

SYNDROME A collection of symptoms (things people complain of) and signs that occur with sufficient frequency to be identified.

TESTES Male sex organs where sperms are produced. Also called testicles or balls.

URETHRITIS Inflammation of the urethra – the tube leading from the urinary bladder to the outside of the body.

Introduction

This book is about diseases that are entirely or often transmitted when people make intimate love. The diseases are sexually transmitted. For a variety of reasons which are discussed in the book, sexually transmitted diseases (STD) are increasing in prevalence. Nearly all are easily cured if an infected person and all his or her sexual partners seek medical help as soon as the person believes she or he has been infected.

The book is to help people learn more about these common diseases. It is divided into three parts. The first is a question and answer section to which you can refer quickly. The second part deals at greater length with each of the diseases. The third part is a brief history of those diseases that were called the venereal diseases in the past.

It might be useful to summarize seven important points about the sexually transmitted diseases. The seven points for thought are:

1

Unless there is a sudden and remarkable change in attitudes towards sexuality, casual sex is likely to continue, and be enjoyed by many men and women.

2

The dangers of casual sex are that the woman may become pregnant and that both sexes may acquire a sexually transmitted disease.

3

Sexually transmitted diseases are infectious diseases, which are spread by sexual intercourse, and should be managed like any other infectious disease. This means that to control the 'worldwide epidemic', all those infected should be treated promptly and properly, and all 'contacts' should be traced so that they may be examined and if found to be infected, may be treated.

4

Any man or woman who develops a discharge from the urethra, painful ulcers or a painless ulcer on the genitals, and who has had sexual intercourse recently should go to a doctor and have tests made.

5

Any person, heterosexual or homosexual, who has sexual intercourse with a number of partners should be examined by a doctor at regular intervals, so that symptomless sexually transmitted diseases, especially gonorrhoea and chlamydia infections, may be detected and treated. In most sexually transmitted diseases, treatment is not painful, nor difficult, but it does need the co-operation of the infected person.

6

There is nothing to be ashamed about in having become infected with a sexually transmitted disease; after all, many eminent men and women have been infected in the past, and may well have been infected recently. What is anti-social, silly and dangerous to the community and to the person, is to avoid going for medical help when the symptoms of the disease occur.

7

A part of the problem is society's attitude to sexuality. So long as sexual intercourse outside marriage continues, and is condemned, and as long as it is considered indecent to talk about the sexually transmitted diseases, so long will they spread and be difficult to control. Education in human sexuality, its delights and its consequences, is needed. This should start in primary schools and continue throughout the school years. It should also continue, through the mass media, so that all citizens may know their responsibilities if they develop a sexually transmitted disease.

1. Questions and answers about sexually transmitted diseases

Non-gonococcal genital infection (NGGI) and chlamydia

What is non-specific genital infection?
This is a sexually transmitted disease often due to a germ called chlamydia, which causes an infection of the man's urethra, and of a woman's cervix. The infection in a man is called non-gonococcal urethritis (NGU). In a woman it is called non-gonococcal genital infection. Usually NGGI causes no symptoms in women; but the infection may spread to the woman's Fallopian tubes, causing pelvic inflammatory disease.

How is NGGI diagnosed?
In a man, a swab taken from the discharge is examined under a microscope, after being stained. Pus cells but no gonococci are seen.

How do you know if you have NGGI?
About 7 to 14 days after sex, a man develops a discharge from the eye of his penis, and may have a burning sensation when he urinates. If he develops the discharge he should go to a doctor, but should avoid passing urine for 2 hours. The doctor takes a swab from the discharge or, if no definite discharge can be seen at the time, may ask him to return the next day with a sample of the first specimen of urine passed.

In most women NGGI causes no symptoms, at least in the early stages of the disease. A few women develop pain in the lower abdomen and/or a smelly vaginal discharge. When examined vaginally by a doctor, pain may be felt deep in the pelvis.

You say that most women infected with NGGI have no symptoms; do any infected men have no symptoms?
A few men whose urethra is infected with non-gonococcal urethritis

(NGU) have no symptoms but may infect their next sexual partner. To avoid this a man who is promiscuous or who has sex with a prostitute should have a swab taken from the urethra and checked.

How is NGGI treated?
The currently favoured treatment is to take a 100 mg tablet of doxycycline (Vibramycin) twice a day with food for 10 days. During this time the person should avoid alcohol. If he or she has sexual intercourse, the man should wear a condom.

Should the man's sexual partners be examined?
They should, as they may have symptomless NGGI.

Is a check-up needed after treatment?
Yes, swabs should be taken to make sure that the person is cured. The reason is that untreated or inadequately treated NGGI or NGU may infect other organs.

What organs are infected?
In men the prostate may be infected initially and the infection may spread further to the eyes, causing conjunctivitis, or to the joints, causing intermittent arthritis. The condition is called Reiter's disease.

In women the infection may cause pelvic inflammatory disease, which may make the woman sterile unless treated.

Gonorrhoea

What is gonorrhoea?
Gonorrhoea is an infectious disease which is sexually transmitted. Most infected people develop an acute infection of the genito-urinary tract, but the person's throat may also be infected if he or she has oral sex.

What causes gonorrhoea?
A small germ called *Neisseria gonorrhoeae* (it is also known as a 'gonococcus'). It is very fragile and dies quickly outside the human body.

How do you know if you have gonorrhoea?
3 to 5 days after sex with an infected person the person's urethra feels uncomfortable or tingles. Very quickly a creamy discharge

appears in the 'eye' of a man's penis, or at the entrance of a woman's urethra. When the person urinates, a burning feeling is felt. The person may also feel off colour. Unfortunately for control of gonorrhoea, over 60 per cent of women (and 20 per cent of men) infected with gonorrhoea have no symptoms.

How is gonorrhoea diagnosed?
A doctor takes a swab from the person's urethra (and in the case of women from the cervix). If the person has had oral sex a throat swab is also taken, while if he or she has had anal sex, a swab is taken from the rectum. The swab is smeared on to a slide which is stained and looked at down a microscope, when the gonococci can be seen. As women may transfer gonococci from the vagina to the rectum, some doctors also take rectal swabs in all suspected cases.

Are any other diagnostic tests made?
If gonorrhoea is found by examining the stained slide, treatment is given. In many clinics, the swab is also smeared on to a culture medium routinely. The culture plate is sent to a laboratory for incubation and examination.

How is gonorrhoea treated?
The person is given tablets or injections of penicillin together with a drug, probenecid, which raises and maintains high levels of penicillin in the blood. Currently the preferred treatment is to give six capsules of amoxycillin and two tablets of probenecid. During treatment alcohol should be avoided. If the throat or rectum are infected, amoxycillin is given in a smaller dose over a three-day period, together with probenecid; or a tablet of doxycycline (Vibramycin) is given every 12 hours, with food, for 6 days.

How do I know if I am cured?
Smears and cultures are taken a week after treatment and examined for gonococci. If no gonococci are found, a man is cured, but a woman should have the test repeated after her next menstrual period before she can be told she is cured. If gonococci are found, the person is given an injection of an antibiotic called spectinomycin.

Can gonorrhoea infect any other organs?
Unfortunately gonorrhoea may spread and infect a woman's Fallo-

pian tubes, causing a pelvic infection. This may damage the tubes so that the woman becomes sterile. In men, untreated gonorrhoea may infect the duct which carries sperm from his testes, and render him sterile. These problems will be avoided if gonorrhoea is diagnosed early and treated adequately.

How can the spread of gonorrhoea be halted?
As nearly all infections occur following sexual intercourse, oral sex or anal sex, an infected person should try to make sure that his or her sexual partner or partners attend a doctor to be checked. As well, any woman or man who has several partners should have a routine check made about every 6 months.

What is resistant gonorrhoea?
Certain strains of gonococci, especially those infecting women in South East Asian countries, are resistant to penicillin, and need to be treated with an injection of spectinomycin.

Are any other diseases transmitted along with gonorrhoea?
Two other diseases may be sexually transmitted at the same time as gonorrhoea. These are chlamydial infection and syphilis. In most cases men are also infected with chlamydia, which causes a discharge from the urethra 2 or 3 weeks after receiving treatment for gonorrhoea. Syphilis may also be transmitted at the same time as gonorrhoea, and people infected with gonorrhoea should have a blood test made 6 weeks after being treated for gonorrhoea.

Genital warts

What are genital warts?
Warts, which look like tiny cauliflowers, appear on a woman's vulva, in her vagina or on her cervix. In a man they appear on his foreskin, on his glans or on the shaft of his penis. The warts may be quite large or almost invisible.

How do genital warts develop?
Warts are caused by a family of viruses, the human papilloma viruses. There are about 30 strains of these viruses which can cause warts on the body. Genital warts are usually caused by strains 6, 16, 18 and 32.

How common are genital warts?
About one sexually active person in 20 has genital warts, but they may be so tiny as to be invisible to the naked eye.

What problems are associated with genital warts?
As well as being unsightly, several strains of the virus may be a factor in the woman developing cervical cancer or the man developing penile cancer.

How are genital warts treated?
A substance called podophyllin is painted carefully on each wart (if there are not too many). The paint is allowed to dry and the patient washes the area an hour later with soap and water. The treatment needs to be repeated several times. The podophyllin kills the wart virus and the wart drops off.

An alternative treatment is to 'vaporize' the warts using a laser, or to burn them with an electric cautery.

Why should genital warts be treated?
Not only are genital warts unsightly, but the wart virus may be a factor in the development of cervical cancer.

Genital herpes

What is herpes?
Herpes is an ancient disease and is caused by a virus. Viruses enter body cells and 'reprogram' them to make multiple copies of the virus which then spreads to other organs. Herpes is caused by two related viruses: *herpes virus 1* which usually causes cold sores; and *herpes virus 2*, which usually causes genital herpes.

What are the symptoms of genital herpes?
Between 5 and 10 days after being infected during sexual intercourse, a small area on the shaft of the penis or the vulva begins to burn or itch. Within 24 hours a crop of reddish bumps appear which blister the next day. Often the area around the blisters becomes swollen, and in women the whole external genitals may swell making urination very painful.

How long does the illness last?
The first attack lasts between 7 and 12 days. The blisters become

ulcers, which are very painful and 'crust' over 4 or 5 days, and then take 3 to 7 days to heal.

Is a person infectious during the attack?
As the ulcers shed large quantities of virus the person is infectious. He or she should wear underpants or panties at night, lest he transfers the virus to his eyes, after scratching the ulcers during sleep. All sexual contact of the genitals should be avoided. If the infected area is touched the person should wash his or her hands carefully.

Does herpes recur?
Unfortunately about 50 per cent of people have a second attack of herpes, and a few (probably less than 5 per cent of people) have recurrent attacks.

Are the recurrent attacks painful?
Usually recurrent herpes is less painful and of shorter duration.

What causes recurrent herpes?
No specific cause has been detected.

Is a person infectious during a recurrent attack?
Yes, sexual contact should be avoided during a recurrent attack.

How does recurrent herpes occur?
During the initial attack, the herpes virus invades the nerve supplying the skin of the infected area. The virus travels along the nerve to a swollen part near the spinal cord, where it lies dormant. It may never be reactivated, or may, when it travels back along the nerve to cause a new crop of blisters.

How is the diagnosis of herpes confirmed?
A swab taken from an ulcer is sent to a virus laboratory.

Is a person who has had herpes likely to infect a sexual partner, when the lesions are absent?
A very few people continue to shed the virus from a previously infected area after the ulcers have healed. However, it is extremely unlikely that the sexual partner will be infected by herpes virus.

Can you catch herpes from a lavatory seat?
Scientists have found that the herpes virus can live for a short time

on a smooth surface at room temperature. They have not established that the virus is able to infect a person during this time. Further, the virus cannot enter the body through the intact skin, which is what comes into contact with the seat.

Does herpes cause cervical cancer?
While there appears to be some association between genital herpes affecting the cervix and the development of cervical cancer 10 to 20 years later, there is no direct evidence, and other factors are more important. However, until the uncertainty is resolved, women who have had genital herpes should have Pap (cervical) smears taken from their cervix every year.

What happens if you have herpes in pregnancy?
About one woman in every 1000 acquires herpes in pregnancy, and about 1 per cent of women have a recurrence of herpes. Genital herpes does not affect the course of pregnancy or the health of the baby until the time of birth. If the mother is shedding herpes virus from her cervix or from a herpes ulcer on her vulva, the baby may acquire herpes during the birth process.

How may herpes affect the newborn baby?
The virus enters the baby's body through his eyes or mouth, and causes a severe illness, shown as herpes hepatitis, pneumonia, brain infections or bleeding problems.

How can this be avoided?
Swabs are taken from the cervix of all women who have acquired herpes during pregnancy or have had an attack of recurrent herpes. The swabs are taken each week or two from the 32nd week. If herpes virus is grown from a swab taken within the two weeks before labour starts, the baby is delivered by caesarean section.

Is there any cure for herpes?
At present there is none, but a drug called acyclovir, which can be applied to the ulcers as an ointment, or given by mouth, reduces the discomfort and shortens the healing time. It is also used to treat babies who have herpes, when it is given intravenously.

Is there any treatment?
Local applications of an analgesic ointment may help, and some

women with severe vulval swelling require to have a catheter placed in the bladder for a few days. Pain killers may also be needed. However, sufferers have a bewildering assortment of remedies which appear to work for some people but have not proved of value in carefully designed trials.

Syphilis

What causes syphilis?
Syphilis is a sexually transmitted disease caused by infection with a tiny corkscrew-shaped germ called *Treponema pallidum* (also called spirochaetes).

What is the chance of catching syphilis if you have sex with an infected person?
One chance in two, if you have sex once; but higher if you have sex several times.

How do I know I have syphilis?
Early syphilis causes a hard-edged ulcer, usually on a man's penis or a woman's vulva, between 3 and 10 weeks after sexual intercourse with an infected person. Occasionally the ulcer – called a chancre – develops on the person's lips after oral sex, or in his or her rectum after anal sex. A few women develop the chancre on the cervix where it cannot be seen but is very infectious. If the penis or vulva is infected, the lymph nodes in the groin become swollen.

How is syphilis diagnosed?
The centre of the ulcer is cleaned and the sides of the ulcer are squeezed by the doctor, until clear fluid wells up from its base. A sample of the fluid is examined under a microscope for the presence of treponemes.

Aren't there blood tests for syphilis?
The blood tests for syphilis are negative for about 6 weeks after infection. After this time the tests become positive. Usually, the VDRL test is made, as a 'screening test', and if it is positive, a further specific test, the FTA–ABS test is made to confirm that the person has syphilis. If syphilis is cured the blood test becomes negative.

Are blood tests made routinely?
In some states in the USA, a blood test is made before the couple can obtain a marriage licence; and in all countries, a blood test is made in early pregnancy.

Why is a blood test made in pregnancy?
Because if the mother has syphilis she may infect her baby which may be born with secondary syphilis.

What is secondary syphilis?
In untreated syphilis the chancre heals in 3 to 4 weeks, but 3 weeks later the person feels ill and may have headaches or joint pains. Then a pale pink skin rash appears which persists for about 6 weeks and slowly fades. A few infected people develop ulcers in the mouth, on the vulva, or in the anus. These lesions usually disappear in 3 to 12 months.

What happens then?
If syphilis is not treated, the third stage may occur 2 to 20 years later. Tertiary syphilis may be associated with painful skin ulcers, gnawing bone pain, damage to the heart, rupture of the main blood vessels, or madness.

How is syphilis treated?
Early syphilis can be cured if the person is given adequate doses of penicillin, either for 10 days or as a single large injection into a muscle. If the person is unable to take penicillin, another antibiotic is chosen.

Must the person continue to be seen?
Yes, follow-up after treatment is essential. Blood tests are made each month for 6 months, and at 9 and 12 months. If the tests are negative by the end of the year the person is cured. On the other hand, the tests may show that further penicillin injections are needed to cure the person.

Can I continue to have sex during this time?
Yes, once the early lesions (the chancre, ulcers or skin rash) have disappeared and an adequate dose of penicillin has been given, sex can be resumed.

How is late syphilis treated?
Late syphilis is treated with large doses of penicillin, but if considerable damage to bones, brain or other organs has occurred the outlook is not good. This is why syphilis should be detected early and treated vigorously.

How can the spread of syphilis be checked?
By making sure that the sexual contacts of every infected person are traced and treated.

AIDS

What is AIDS?
The word is an acronym for Acquired Immune Deficiency Syndrome and is due to a defect in the person's protective immune system, which renders him (or her) more likely to develop a severe, often fatal, infection.

Who gets AIDS?
Homosexual and bisexual men are most often infected, followed by drug abusers (who mainline); Haitians; and others.

How is AIDS caused?
AIDS is caused by a virus called the human immunodeficiency virus (HIV). The virus is transmitted by sexual intercourse and a person is more likely to be infected after anal intercourse than after vaginal intercourse. Usually the infected person has no symptoms for 2 or 3 years, but can infect others. After this time he or she develops symptoms and has AIDS.

What causes AIDS?
AIDS is caused by a virus – the human immunodeficiency virus (HIV), which is usually sexually transmitted. About 80 per cent of people who have been at higher risk for several years of being infected (homosexual and bisexual men who have several partners, and intravenous drug users who share needles) have become infected as judged by a test for HIV.

Many people infected with the AIDS virus (HIV) remain healthy for some time, but over a period of 5 to 8 years about half of them will develop the AIDS Related Complex or full-blown AIDS, and over a 15-year period up to 75 per cent will develop full-blown AIDS. Those people who have been infected but who are healthy may infect others with whom they have sex, particularly anal sex, or if their blood is transferred to another person, usually by sharing a needle.

How do you know if you have AIDS?
The less severe form, known as the Aids Related Complex (ARC) is associated with symptoms that have lasted for 3 months at least and include one or more of:

1. Fever and night sweats.
2. Swollen lymph nodes in at least three places.
3. Weight loss.
4. Chronic diarrhoea.
5. A low white cell count in the blood.

This form is only rarely fatal. Over a period of time about three-quarters of people who have the Aids Related Complex will develop full-blown AIDS.

What is the chance of dying from AIDS?
The mild form is only rarely fatal, but 75 per cent of people infected go on to develop a severe form. The severe form is more serious and most of those infected die within 2 years.

What is the risk of catching AIDS?
If you practise safe sex, by making sure that the man wears a condom throughout sexual intercourse, and you are not an intravenous drug user who shares needles, the risk is negligible.

How can AIDS be avoided?
It is not known for certain, but multiple partners and anal intercourse may be factors. The fewer partners and the less anal intercourse the less the risk. In addition drug abusers should avoid 'mainlining'.

Myths about AIDS
You can't get AIDS from casual contact with an infected person. Shaking hands, hugging, crying, coughing, or sneezing will not spread AIDS. Nor will social kissing, sharing food or swimming in a

pool which has been used by a person infected with HIV. Now that all blood donors are carefully screened you will not get AIDS from a blood transfusion, or from an injection of the hepatitis B vaccine.

Sexually transmitted vaginal infections

What are sexually transmitted vaginal infections?
Three main vaginal infections occur which may be transmitted sexually but often are not. These are candidiasis (vaginal monilia, vaginal thrush); trichomoniasis; and 'non-specific' vaginitis.

How does a woman know if she has a vaginal infection?
First she develops a vaginal discharge, which may have a fishy smell and may cause itching or burning. However, these symptoms may occur when a woman has an increase in the normal vaginal moisture. For this reason she should visit a doctor.

What should the doctor do?
It is impossible to differentiate between an excessive normal discharge and vaginal infections, or between the various infections, by looking at the vagina or at the discharge.

The doctor must take a swab from the discharge. He may decide to examine the swab by smearing it on a slide in his office or surgery, or he may place it in a 'culture medium' and send it to a laboratory.

What is candidiasis?
This is a vaginal infection caused by a fungus. In some cases the woman's partner develops an itchy penis, which is why candidiasis is included as a sexually transmitted disease.

How is candida diagnosed?
By looking at a stained slide when the threads and blobs of the fungus can be seen.

How is candida treated?
The woman places a tablet (called an ovule) of an antifungal drug high in her vagina for one or three nights. She may also apply an antifungal ointment to her vulva, if it is itchy. Her partner should apply the ointment to his penis if it is itchy.

Should I return for follow-up treatment?
It is wise, but not essential, to have a further swab taken 7 to 10 days after the treatment is concluded.

What is trichomoniasis?
This is a vaginal infection caused by a tiny one-celled parasite. It is often sexually transmitted.

How is trichomoniasis diagnosed?
A portion of the discharge is mixed with a drop of saline and observed through a microscope, when the parasite can be seen moving through the mixture. Occasionally a culture is made, and after incubation the parasite is looked for.

How is trichomoniasis treated?
The person and his or her partner takes a drug called metronidazole three times a day for 7 days or, if preferred, a related drug called tinidazole as a single dose of 4 tablets. Alcohol must be avoided for the duration of the treatment, plus one day, because it may lead to nausea, vomiting and abdominal cramps.

What is 'non-specific' vaginitis (amine vaginosis)?
This is a vaginal infection due to the interaction of two types of germ in the vagina. The interaction causes a greyish vaginal discharge, which has a fishy smell due to the release of amines.

How is amine vaginosis treated?
The treatment is the same as that for trichomoniasis.

Hepatitis B

Why is hepatitis B considered a sexually transmitted disease?
Some people who have had hepatitis and recovered continue to excrete the hepatitis virus into their gut. These people are called carriers. If another person has close body contact and particularly anal or oral sex with them, the infection may spread.

Can carriers be detected?
Carriers have a marker in their blood called hepatitis B surface antigen. This can be detected by a blood test.

Who are most likely to be carriers?
About 15 per cent of South East Asians, 10 per cent of promiscuous homosexual men and 8 per cent of drug addicts are carriers.

How can the partner of a carrier avoid getting hepatitis B?
He or she should avoid anal or oral sex until he has been given hepatitis B vaccine injections.

Pubic lice

How do you get crab (pubic) lice?
Lice cannot jump and are transferred during close sexual encounters. They attach themselves to pubic hairs, and lay their eggs in the skin.

What are the symptoms of pubic lice infections?
Itching of the skin beneath the pubic hair and occasionally some blood after scratching.

How are pubic lice treated?
By applying a shampoo of 0.5% malathion or gamma benzene hexachloride (Gamene, Lorexane, Quellada) to the skin, and while it is still wet combing the area carefully with a fine-toothed metal comb. An alternative treatment is to leave the malathion or gamma benzene on the hairy area for 24 hours and then shower or have a bath.

Rare sexually transmitted diseases

CHANCROID

What is chancroid?
It is a sexually transmitted disease, usually occurring in the tropics, and is caused by a small organism.

What are the symptoms of chancroid?
3 to 7 days after sex with an infected person, painful pimples occur on the man's penis or the woman's labia. They grow rapidly and ulcerate, causing soft, painful, multiple ulcers. The lymph nodes in the groin also become swollen.

How is chancroid diagnosed?
A swab is taken from the ulcer, which is stained and examined under a microscope.

What is the treatment of chancroid?
Sulphonamides cure the disease.

Should I attend for follow-up after cure?
Yes. When chancroid was acquired, you might also have caught syphilis. The incubation period for syphilis is long, so that you should attend for a check-up if you develop a sore on the genitals, or a reddish skin rash which persists for more than 14 days. You should also have a blood test for syphilis.

LYMPHOGRANULOMA VENEREUM (LGV)

What is LGV?
LGV is a sexually transmitted disease due to an organism that resembles chlamydia. It is very rare in Europe but more common in Africa.

What are the symptoms of LGV?
7 to 12 days after sex with an infected person an ulcer develops on the penis of a man or on a woman's vulva. At the same time the nodes in the groin become enlarged, rubbery and covered by a shiny reddish skin. The ulcer heals slowly and the nodes in the groin either heal or break down, discharging cheesy pus through ragged holes in the skin.

How is LGV treated?
By giving an antibiotic called doxycycline (Vibramycin).

GRANULOMA INGUINALE

What is granuloma inguinale?
It is a rare sexually transmitted disease which requires repeated contact for infection to be transferred.

What causes granuloma inguinale?
A bacterium with an unpronounceable name!

What are the symptoms?
After an interval of days, weeks or months, ragged ulcers appear on the genitals which spread to affect most of the genitals unless treated.

How is it diagnosed?
By taking a swab from the ulcer.

How is it treated?
By giving a course of antibiotics.

2. The problem of sexually transmitted diseases today

Information obtained from many nations of the world by the World Health Organization confirms that, in the past 15 years, the number of people infected with a sexually transmitted disease has been increasing. The increase applies to the three sexually transmitted diseases that constitute, in law, the venereal diseases, but more particularly to other sexually transmitted diseases. For example, in many countries a sexually transmitted infection of the genitals called non-gonococcal genital infection (NGGI) is more common than gonorrhoea. As the disease in men usually infects the urethra, it is also called non-gonococcal urethritis (NGU). Another widely publicized example of an increasing incidence of a sexually transmitted disease is that of genital herpes.

The legally notifiable venereal diseases – gonorrhoea, syphilis and chancroid – obtained their name from Venus, the goddess of love. Since the organisms which cause the diseases usually enter the body during sexual intercourse with an infected person, the term was a useful one. But the increasing prevalence of other sexually transmitted diseases and the odium attached to the term 'venereal disease' suggest that the designation is now archaic, and the diseases should be called sexually transmitted diseases. It must be realized that the sexual contact that leads to the spread of the disease may be orogenital or anal as well as during sexual intercourse in which the man's penis is inserted into the woman's vagina.

It is impossible to be sure how many people acquire a sexually transmitted infection in any year. Sample surveys in the USA, Britain and Australia, to name only three countries, show that fewer than 10 per cent of cases of NGU or of gonorrhoea treated by doctors in private practice are reported to the authorities. The reporting of syphilis is also low: only 30 to 50 per cent of treated cases are reported, although, in law, doctors have an obligation to make a report to the health authorities. The World Health Organization believes that of the legally notifiable sexually transmitted diseases, gonorrhoea infects more than 200 million people each year, and that syphilis is detected in over 50 million people each year. Genital herpes is only notifiable in some countries. The hysteria occasioned by magazine and newspaper 'scare-mongering' in 1981–3 in the USA, suggested that an 'epidemic' of herpes had occurred. There is no evidence for this. In fact herpes may be less common than gonorrhoea and four times as many cases of genital warts occur each year.

In view of the high incidence of many sexually transmitted diseases, doctors who diagnose them have a moral, if not legal, obligation to try to induce the patient to disclose the name of any sexual partner or partners he or she may have had, so that they may be screened and, if infected, treated.

Sexually transmitted diseases are infectious and contagious. This means that they are transferred easily from an infected person to a non-infected person by close bodily contact. The only difference between the sexually transmitted diseases and other contagious diseases is that in the former the contact is of a sexual nature. You cannot acquire an STD from a lavatory seat! In most societies sexual intercourse is not discussed openly, and infection acquired during sexual contact is thought by society, and by the infected person, to be disgusting, indecent and something to be concealed. The control of an infectious disease depends on treating the infected person and in tracing infected contacts so that they may be treated. The purpose of informing the health authorities that a person has contracted gonorrhoea or syphilis is to enable them to do just this; and patients or their doctors who refuse to co-operate – as all too many do – are encouraging the spread of the diseases.

Unfortunately, ignorance and prejudice about sexually transmitted diseases are widespread and some doctors may be as ignorant as is the general public. Some doctors show attitudes of disapproval and condemnation when a patient, who thinks he or she may have a sexually transmitted disease, seeks advice. Some patients, particularly young people who are increasingly being infected, are apprehensive, fearful and ashamed to seek help in case the doctor is critical and disapproving. Because of this they may conceal the disease in the hope that the symptoms will go away. They often do, but unfortunately the individual continues to be infectious to any subsequent sexual partner.

Many myths have arisen because the diseases are not discussed openly. This disapproving attitude to the sexually transmitted diseases extends to the type of clinic where advice and treatment are given. All too often it is an ugly building, difficult to find, unpleasant to attend, uncomfortable to wait in, dirty and dingy. As the acquisition of a sexually transmitted disease carries a marked social stigma, many possible patients are reluctant to attend for treatment, and many an anxious patient is deterred when he or she sees the inadequate facilities. This reticence would be overcome to some extent if the clinics were in well-appointed and pleasant buildings, in convenient areas, open at convenient times, where first-class treatment was given, where the patient knew he or she would be treated confidentially without any moral strictures being passed, and where all treatment was free.

The sexually transmitted diseases can conveniently be divided into three groups (Table 2/1):

1. The major diseases which, if untreated, may damage body organs unconnected with the genital tract.
2. The minor diseases which are usually localized to the genital tract and have no damaging long-term effects.
3. The rare sexually transmitted diseases which are usually acquired in the tropics and which cause damage outside the genital tract.

Nothing of what I have written so far explains why there has been such a considerable upsurge in the venereal diseases in recent years. It is a strange paradox that the increase has occurred at a time when, in so many nations, affluence has never been greater, education is widespread, and the treatment for sexually transmitted disease is painless and effective.

The principal reason for the increase seems to be an increasingly 'permissive' attitude to sexuality. If no individual ever had sexual intercourse, except with the partner he or she had married, the diseases would almost certainly be eradicated. As this situation has never applied in the whole history of mankind (except perhaps in the

Table 2/1 Sexually transmitted diseases

THE MAJOR SEXUALLY TRANSMITTED DISEASES
(in order of frequency of infection reported annually)

* Non-gonococcal genital infection (including non-gonococcal urethritis and chlamydia infection)
* Gonorrhoea
* Genital warts
* Genital herpes
* Syphilis

DISEASES THAT ARE OFTEN TRANSMITTED SEXUALLY

* AIDS (human immunodeficiency virus, HIV)
* Viral hepatitis

THE MINOR SEXUALLY TRANSMITTED DISEASES

* Vaginal candidiasis (monilia or thrush)
* Vaginal trichomoniasis
* Non-specific vaginal infection (amine vaginosis)
* Pubic lice
* Molluscum contagiosum

THE RARE SEXUALLY TRANSMITTED DISEASES

* Chancroid
* Lymphogranuloma venereum
* Granuloma inguinale

garden of Eden) it is entirely unrealistic to expect it to happen now. Human sexuality is a deep and forceful drive which most people need to overcome by embarking on a sexual relationship. It is also influenced by fashion, and when fashion adopts an increased 'permissiveness' in sexual relations, sexually transmitted diseases are likely to spread.

For several centuries in Western societies there has been a double standard of sexuality. Young men, if not encouraged, at least were not discouraged, or disapproved of, when they copulated. Young women were meant to remain chaste until marriage. But for young men to copulate they had to have partners, who were usually female. Some of them had a sexually transmitted disease and infected the young men, who in turn infected the chaste young women after marriage.

In recent years many young women have rejected this double

standard and have joined the ranks of those who have sex. In recent years there has been more casual sex, and an increase in sexual activity by young people.

Studies in Britain, Scandinavia and the USA show that by the age of 20, a majority of young men and women have had sexual intercourse. In most cases the sexual relationship is on a one-to-one basis, but at least one-fifth of sexually active teenagers have several partners. They have been called 'sexual adventurers' and as such are at greater risk of contracting a sexually transmitted disease than 'serial monogamists'.

A further factor in the increasing sexual activity of teenagers is the falling age at which a woman reaches menarche, the onset of menstruation, and becomes sexually desirable and receptive. One hundred years ago the median age of menarche was 17, today it has fallen to 13. This has led to a longer period between menarche and marriage. During this time sexual experimentation has become more common. However, it would be fallacious to see an increase in sexual permissiveness as a phenomenon of the late twentieth century. Premarital sexual intercourse was common in nineteenth-century Europe, particularly in rural areas and in the slums of the grimy industrial cities.

What distinguishes the present time is that with reduced mortality there are many more teenagers who talk openly about their sexual experiences and who are much more mobile. In addition, social and societal changes (often by the parents of teenagers) have led to sub-groups of adolescents who are at a considerable risk of acquiring a sexually transmitted disease, according to a respected Danish physician, Dr Ekstrom.

These are the disaffected teenagers who congregate in the larger cities and sell their bodies to obtain money for drugs and excitement. They have poor relationships with their parents, they often come from broken homes, they have frequent changes of schools and jobs and, obviously, sexual partners. They are no less intelligent than other teenagers. Dr Ekstrom believes that additional education in the social aspects of life is needed in schools, and more importantly there is need to improve social conditions for the at-risk group. He stresses that the management of sexually transmitted diseases is not only a matter of diagnosis and treatment: it is a social problem and requires a medico-social solution. The Danish experience is being mirrored increasingly in all large cities.

The increased sexual activity of women has had a further effect. Women who are infected with NGGI infection or with gonorrhoea often have no symptoms (as do a few men), or such mild symptoms that they ignore them. But they are infectious and they may infect their next sexual partners for weeks or months or even years. In two large series of patients, reported from Britain and the USA, between 50 and 80 per cent of women diagnosed as having gonorrhoea were completely symptomless and only attended the hospital because they had been asked to do so by their infected sexual partner. This large 'reservoir' of women with symptomless, silent gonorrhoea is one reason for its spread, particularly if the infected woman is sexually active with several partners. In other words, if she is promiscuous.

The spread of sexually transmitted diseases has been encouraged by the increasing mobility of people who seek work in places often far away from their homes. Many European countries have sought foreign-born workers to man their factories. These men, who are usually young and single, come from the poorer nations of Southern Europe, North Africa and West Asia. They tend to live in groups in the larger industrial cities. They are frequently bored and lonely, and find transient companionship and contact with local young women in clubs and pubs. The young women are often emotionally unstable, sexually active and infected with symptomless gonorrhoea, NGGI or untreated syphilis.

Britain, in the 1960s, accepted large numbers of immigrants from the Caribbean, Pakistan and India. These migrants, like the migrant workers of Europe, concentrated in the larger industrial cities where there was a better chance of finding work, and where they could mix more readily with people from their homelands. Like the European migrant workers they sought companionship in clubs and pubs and, as in Europe, local young women were sexually willing, sexually able and often infected. So the sexually transmitted diseases spread. This led to the myth, still firmly believed by many English people, that the coloured migrants brought 'venereal diseases' with them. The evidence is that the majority of migrants obtained their infection from local women and were uninfected when they arrived in Britain. This has led to one British authority, Dr Morton, to state, 'My own experience is that much more infection is imported by UK-born tourists returning from the Continent than by immigrants.'

The increased opportunity people have to travel, either alone or in 'package tours', has also increased the spread of the sexually transmitted diseases. Away from home, free from the constraints of a familiar environment, warm with sun and alcohol, relaxed and sedated, the holiday-maker sees casual copulation not only as sensible but pleasurable and desirable. And to meet the demand, a supply of local women (and men) is available. Many have either gonorrhoea, NGGI (often due to chlamydia) or infectious syphilis. The evidence that these casual encounters lead to an increase in the sexually transmitted diseases is demonstrated by figures from Sweden and Holland which show that 20 per cent of all cases of infectious syphilis diagnosed in 1975 was imported by returning tourists, or by businessmen. Yet when these people return home, they are all to ready to criticize the 'permissive' young while ignoring their own sexual activities.

Other studies have shown that merchant sailors and members of the Armed Forces are particularly likely to be infected with sexually transmitted diseases and to infect others. Deprived of female company for long periods and relatively rich when they reach a port, they are particularly susceptible to advances by local prostitutes or enthusiastic amateur fornicators. The high incidence of a particularly resistant strain of gonorrhoea acquired by the US servicemen in Vietnam, and passed gratuitously to women in countries as far apart as Australia and Austria, is an example of this. Men or women who are itinerant, such as commercial travellers, cane cutters, pea pickers, transient workers, and particularly lorry drivers, have a higher than average risk of acquiring and spreading a sexually transmitted disease.

In several studies homosexuality has been implicated in the spread of sexually transmitted diseases. These studies refer to male homosexuals, who are claimed to be particularly promiscuous. The studies have been made in cities where promiscuous homosexuals gather. The results refer to these men, who frequent homosexual meeting places and who often have one-night stands at frequent intervals. The casually encountered sexual partner, or the man who is 'cruising', may have symptomless gonorrhoeal infection or syphilitic infection of his anus, or may have infectious gonorrhoea of his genitals. Oro-genital or anal intercourse permits the disease to be transmitted.

The reports suggest that a much higher than expected number of homosexuals compared with heterosexuals acquire one of the sexually transmitted diseases. The higher rates have been reported from London, Amsterdam, Sydney, New York and San Francisco.

What is not clear is whether these homosexuals are sexually promiscuous because of an emotional defect, or whether their promiscuity is due to society's reaction to homosexuality and the fear many homosexuals have of being condemned, criticized and even prosecuted if they form a permanent relationship with another man. It must also be stressed that promiscuous homosexuals who congregate in large cities, frequenting gay bars and bath houses, constitute fewer than 5 per cent of all homosexuals. The majority of homosexual men, who form at least 5 per cent of the male population, live quiet unobtrusive lives, usually in a one-to-one relationship, and change partners as infrequently as most heterosexual males.

In all nations, whether in the rich, affluent, developed third of the world, or in the hungry, developing two-thirds of the world, there is a drift to the cities. This has been going on for the past 50 years but is currently gathering momentum. One calculation suggests that by AD 2000, only 15 years from now, over 80 per cent of people in the developed nations and over 55 per cent of people in the developing nations will live in towns. Many of those migrating to escape the boredom and rigidity of village life are single, young and anxious to throw off the contraints of their old life. They are likely to seek solace, when lonely, with city girls, some of whom will certainly be infected with a sexually transmitted disease.

Many will have sex with prostitutes, either street-walkers or in a brothel. Although the latter may have monthly medical checks made on the premises, some of the women are likely to have acquired NGGI or gonorrhoea, between the checks and may transmit the infection to their clients. A study in Sydney, Australia, in 1983 showed that in one brothel 10 per cent of the women had gonorrhoea in spite of medical checks. To overcome this problem the National Venereology Council of Australia recommended that weekly medical checks should be made, and clients should wear condoms. Sex with a street-walker is more dangerous, as these women rarely have medical checks and often continue to have sex when they know they have a sexually transmitted disease.

Those who have followed the argument this far will appreciate that there is no single cause for the accelerating increase in sexually transmitted diseases which have become, in the words of the World Health Organization 'a world-wide epidemic'. The sexually transmitted diseases infect people of all classes, all professions and all races. All that is needed is to have sexual intercourse with an infected partner.

The statistics do show an increase in the frequency of the disease in teenagers, and especially teenage girls, but no age is exempt. Men are twice as likely to be infected as women, but this is merely because men copulate casually more often than women. It is true, as Dr Catterall writes, that 'In the final analysis the problem is a moral one and depends upon the standards of sexual behaviour which prevail in the community as a whole.' Promiscuity results in the spread of sexually transmitted diseases and they cannot be contracted if risks of infection are not taken. But this statement is no help, for casual sexual intercourse is not prevented by exhortation, nor was it in the periods of history that were apparently sexually repressive.

What is needed is realism. Most people are not going to change their attitudes to their own sexuality, and many are going to continue to have casual sexual intercourse, whatever moralists say. An increasing number of people believe that sexual intercourse between consenting adults, whether hetero- or homosexual, is a personal matter and should not be interfered with by society. Society must recognize these facts and, rather than condemn silently, must attempt to reduce the dangers of promiscuity. These dangers are unwanted pregnancies and the spread of the sexually transmitted diseases.

In part, the change will come through education; in part through the change in the attitude of the opinion-makers, and the leaders of society, towards sexually transmitted diseases.

Since human sexuality is such a deep, instinctive drive, knowledge of human sexuality and its consequences should form part of the education of every individual. I believe that education in human sexuality, including sexual responsibility, should extend throughout the school years, starting at the age of 8 or 9. Factual knowledge about the sexually transmitted diseases should have been given, and discussions held in mixed classes, before children reach puberty. This educational experience may deter some from later casual sex, and induce those who wish to be promiscuous to seek medical help without fear or shame, should they develop a sexually transmitted disease. Whether education alone will reduce the incidence of sexually transmitted diseases will be shown only by experience. It will not increase casual sexuality, or 'harm the fabric of society', as certain conservatives believe. The evidence from Scandinavia is clear on this point.

The spread of the sexually transmitted diseases will only be arrested if each person with whom an infected individual has had sexual intercourse is contacted, examined and, if infected, treated. In most Western countries, the traditional method of 'contact tracing', in cases of the legally notifiable diseases, is for the doctor who treats the person to hand him, or her, a contact slip or slips to give to his sexual partner or partners, asking them to go to a hospital or to a private doctor, taking the slips with them. This method has not been very successful, particularly among the 90 per cent of patients who seek private treatment from a private doctor. Increasing numbers of people believe that contacts should be sought by specially trained social workers who could more readily persuade them to be examined and, if needed, to be treated. This method seems to have worked in the USSR, where an efficient service has been established. The names of all patients who have contracted venereal disease, and their known sexual partners, are compulsorily (but confidentially) notified to special health workers, who make the contacts. In the USSR the incidence of venereal disease is declining, at a time when it is rising in the other developed nations.

Whether compulsion will be needed in other nations is uncertain, but there is no reason why the public should object. They do not object to the compulsory notification of diphtheria, poliomyelitis, typhoid fever or other infectious diseases. The acceptance of compulsory notification and contact tracing by trained and carefully selected health workers would be more readily accepted if the public's inaccurate understanding of the nature of the sexually transmitted diseases was improved by using the media to educate them imaginatively.

A campaign should also be initiated using radio, television and magazines to induce high-risk groups, particularly promiscuous homosexual men, and prostitutes, to seek voluntary examinations at regular intervals.

From the point of view of the individual who is at risk of catching a sexually transmitted disease, what should be done? The purpose of the book is to explain just this. But any person who, after sexual intercourse, is concerned that he or she has acquired a sexually transmittable disease, should visit a doctor or a hospital so that tests can be made and should not be afraid or ashamed to make a visit.

Because so many women infected with gonorrhoea have no knowledge that they have the disease, any woman who has multiple sexual partners should have an examination periodically. She should neither be fearful nor ashamed, for her sexuality is her own affair and the only function of the doctor is to detect and treat a possible infection.

A question that may be asked is: what are the chances of my getting one of the diseases if I have casual sexual intercourse with an infected partner? This is very difficult to determine, but the evidence is that five out of every ten people, whether male or female, acquire gonorrhoea if they have sexual intercourse with an infected partner. And about one in every two people who have intercourse with a partner who has active syphilis will develop syphilis. These figures apply to a single casual episode of sexual intercourse. Repeated sexual intercourse with an infected partner makes it much more likely that you will catch the disease. Information about the infectiousness of the other sexually transmitted diseases is not available although it is known that genital herpes is highly infectious when the blisters are present.

As well as these measures, medical research is urgently needed. Science has devised and produced vaccination against poliomyelitis, diphtheria, whooping-cough, rubella, measles, typhoid and small pox, among others. If funds were made available it should be possible to develop vaccines against gonorrhoea, herpes, non-gonococcal urethritis and syphilis within a short time. It is true that the threat to society by the spread of the HIV (AIDS) virus has led to considerable funds being made available for research to find a cure for AIDS. However, funds are needed for research in to the other more common, but less lethal, sexually transmitted diseases.

Until vaccines are developed to protect an individual against these diseases, the only protection is to practise safer sex. Safe sex implies that people limit the number of the sexual partners, preferably to one, and if they choose to have casual sex that the man wears a condom.

It is an odd comment about the priorities of society that vast sums can be expended on space exploration but that, largely because of the limitation of funds, no scientific group has developed vaccines which will eliminate gonorrhoea or NGGI, each of which last year infected at least 200 million people; genital herpes which probably recurrently affects 100 million people; or syphilis, which infected 50 million. Twenty-five years ago an American authority, Dr Knox, speaking in Denver, Colorado, said wryly that if as much money was put into venereal disease research as went into research into poliomyelitis, which neither cripples nor kills as many people, a vaccine would be found in a few years.

Psychological aspects of STDs

These public health aspects of STDs are only one aspect of the problem. Equally important is the individual's reaction to having been infected. Some infected people believe that the infection is a deserved consequence of their sexual behaviour and is a punishment for having 'sinned' sexually. Other infected persons believe that they have been unlucky in becoming infected because they were unfortunate enough to come into contact with a particularly virulent germ. At the other end of the scale, some people believe that having been infected is a matter of pride and signifies that they are 'macho'. Exploration of these myths is needed to ensure that the person will comply with treatment and hopefully will change certain 'high risk' sexual behaviours.

The process of this exploration includes counselling.

COUNSELLING

Many people who are diagnosed as having a sexually transmitted disease are devastated psychologically, at least for a time. This concern has increased since the AIDS epidemic.

These people need help and should be able to obtain counselling. Counselling means that they can talk with an informed health professional or other skilled person about the options available to them, and how they may better comply with the proposed treatment and may avoid a further infection.

Counselling includes helping the person obtain additional information about the disease so that his or her psychological damage is reduced and the person feels better about himself or herself.

In the interaction with a non-judgemental, warm, empathetic counsellor the person's sexual preferences and behaviours may need to be explored. For example, in a study reported from an STD clinic in London, 20 per cent of infected white women reported engaging in anal sex, which led to investigations which otherwise would not have been made, and to a modification of treatment. The purpose of counselling is to help the infected person to become more aware of the nature of the infection, and of his or her reaction to it, so that questions that trouble him or her may be answered, myths demolished and avoidance of a further infection increased.

3. Female and male

In the great majority of instances the organisms that cause the sexually transmitted diseases gain entry to the human body through the genitals. In a few cases the organism which causes syphilis – the *Treponema pallidum* – is transferred from the mother's blood to that of the unborn baby through the afterbirth. Sometimes a woman, or a homosexual man, is infected on the tongue or lips when sucking the infected penis of a sexual partner. Sometimes a man may be infected in a similar way by kissing an infected woman's vulval area.

The organisms that cause non-specific genital infection and gonorrhoea may spread from the place of entry in women to invade other organs which make up the genital tract. Men, too, may experience spread of gonorrhoea to affect their internal genital organs, or their testes. In addition, the organisms that cause the most common sexually transmitted disease in men, non-gonococcal urethritis, may spread to affect other genital organs.

A knowledge of the anatomy of the genital organs is important if the sexually transmitted diseases are to be understood fully.

Woman

The anatomical name for the area of the external genitals in the female is the vulva. It is made up of several structures which surround the entrance to the vagina, and each of which has its own separate function (Fig. 3/1). The labia majora (or the large lips of the vagina) are two large folds of skin which contain sweat glands and hair follicles embedded in fat. The size of the labia majora varies considerably. In infancy and in old age they are small and the fat is not present; in the reproductive years, between puberty and menopause, they are well filled with fatty tissue. In front (looked at from

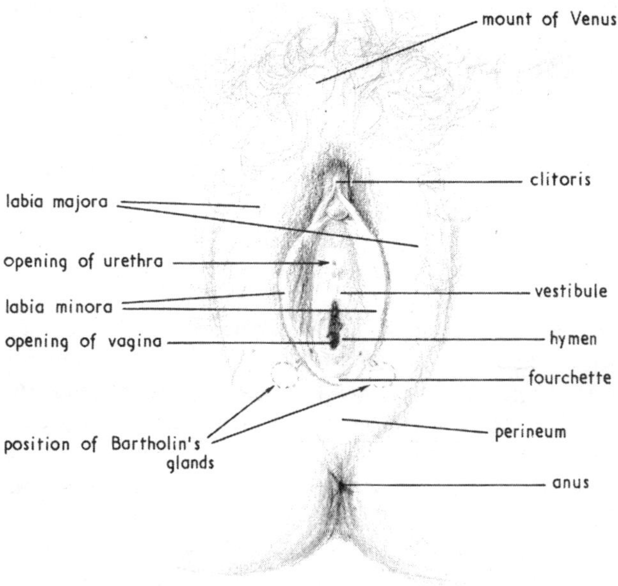

Fig. 3/1 The external genitals of a virgin

between the legs), they join together in the pad of fat that surmounts the pubic bone, and which was called the 'mount of Venus' (mons veneris) by the ancient anatomists when they noted it was most developed in the reproductive years.

Both the labia and more particularly the mons veneris, are covered with hair, the quantity of which varies from woman to woman. The pubic hair on the abdominal side of the mons veneris terminates in a straight line, while in the male the hair stretches upwards in an inverted 'V' to reach the umbilicus. The inner surfaces of the labia majora are free from hair and are separated by a small groove from the thin labia minora, which guard the entrance to the vagina. The organism that causes syphilis may be transferred during sexual intercourse from an ulcer on the penis of the infected man and, entering through a tiny, invisible abrasion, may form an ulcer on the inner surface of one or other of the labia majora.

The labia minora (the small lips) are delicate folds of skin which contain a little fatty tissue. They vary in size and it was once believed that large labia minora were due to masturbation, which at that time was considered evil. It is now known that this is nonsense. In front, the labia minora split into two folds, one of which passes over, and the other under, the clitoris, and at the back they join to form the fourchette, which is always torn during childbirth. In the reproductive years, the labia minora are hidden by the enlarged labia majora but in childhood and old age the labia minora appear more prominent because the labia majora are relatively small.

The clitoris is the exact female equivalent of the male penis. The fold of the labia minora that passes over it is equivalent to the male foreskin (prepuce). It covers and protects the clitoris. The fold that passes under it is equivalent to the small band of tissue which joins the pink glans of the penis to the skin which covers it. It is called the frenulum. The clitoris is made up of erectile tissue, which fills with blood during sexual excitement. It is extremely sensitive to the touch. Orgasm in women occurs by the indirect stimulation of the clitoris by the movement of the penis in the vagina in sexual intercourse. It also occurs if the clitoris is gently stroked with the fingers or licked with the partner's tongue. The clitoris varies considerably in size, but is usually that of a green pea; as sexual excitement mounts, it increases in size. Once again this varies considerably between individuals.

The cleft below the clitoris and between the labia minora is called the vestibule (or entrance). Just below the clitoris is the external opening of that part of the urinary tract (the urethra) which connects the bladder to the outside world. The urethra in a woman is quite short, and several small side tubes, called Skene's ducts, open into it. The lining membrane of the urethra and its ducts is thin and delicate. It is through this thin membrane that the germs causing gonorrhoea enter the body, being transferred during sexual intercourse from an infected partner. The tubes that form Skene's ducts are complex in shape, and if the gonococcus gets into these the infection can linger for a long time, unless it is adequately treated. In a woman this may be without any symptoms, but she is able to give gonorrhoea to any man with whom she has sexual intercourse.

Below the external urethral orifice is the hymen, which surrounds the vaginal orifice. The hymen is a thin, incomplete fold of membrane, which has one or more apertures in it. It varies considerably in shape and in elasticity, but is generally stretched or torn during the first attempt at sexual intercourse (Fig. 3/2). The tearing is usually followed by a small amount of bleeding.

In many cultures the rupture of the hymen (also called the maidenhead), and the consequent bleed, were considered to be the sign that the girl was a virgin at the time of marriage, and the bed was inspected on the morning after the first night of the honeymoon for evidence of blood. Although an 'intact' hymen is considered a sign of virginity, it is not a reliable sign, because in some cases coitus fails to cause a tear, and in others the hymen may have been torn previously by exploring fingers, either of the woman herself or of a consort. The stretching and tearing of the hymen at the first attempt at sexual intercourse may be painful, particularly if the partners are apprehensive or ignorant of sexual matters. If the couple are well adjusted, the discomfort is minimal. Childbirth causes a much greater tearing of the hymen and after delivery only a few tags remain. They are called carunculae myrtiformes (Fig. 3/2). Just outside the hymen, still within the vestibule but deep beneath the skin, are two collections of

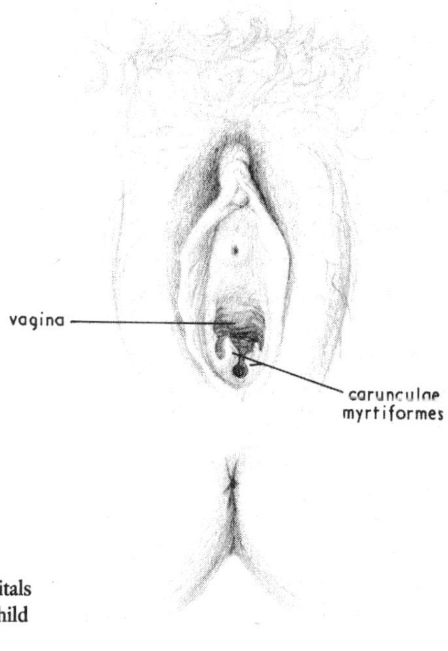

Fig. 3/2 The external genitals of a woman who has had a child

erectile tissue which fill with blood during sexual arousal. Deep in the backward part of the vestibule are two pea-sized glands which also secrete fluid during sexual arousal and moisten the entrance to the vagina, so that the penis may more readily enter it without discomfort. These glands occasionally become infected. They are known as Bartholin's glands. Like the urethra, Bartholin's glands are lined with a thin, delicate membrane. Once again, the organisms causing gonorrhoea may enter a woman's body by invading Bartholin's glands.

The part of the vulva between the posterior fourchette and the anus, and the muscles that lie under the skin, form a pyramid-shaped wedge of tissue separating the vagina and the rectum. It is called the perineum, and is of considerable importance in childbirth.

The vagina is a muscular tube which stretches upwards and backwards from the vestibule to reach the uterus. As well as being muscular, it contains a well-developed network of veins which become distended in sexual arousal. Normally the walls of the vagina lie close together, the vagina being a potential cavity which is distended by intravaginal tampons during menstruation, by the penis during sexual intercourse and by the infant during childbirth, when it stretches very considerably to permit the baby to be born. The vagina is about 9cm (3¾in) long and at the upper end the cervix, or neck, of the uterus projects into it (Fig. 3/3). The vagina lies between the bladder in front and the rectum (or back passage) behind. At the sides it is surrounded and protected by the strong muscles of the floor of the pelvis.

Unless the vagina has been damaged, injured or tightened at operation, or has not developed owing to an absence of sex hormones, its size is quite adequate for sexual intercourse. A woman who menstruates has a normal-sized vagina, and 'difficulty' at intercourse is not due to her being 'small-made'. This is a myth. The cause lies not in the vagina, but in a mental fear of sexual intercourse which leads the woman to tighten the muscles that support the vagina to such an extent that coitus is painful.

The vagina is a remarkable organ. Not only is it capable of great distension, but it keeps itself clean. The cells that form its walls are 30 cells deep, lying on each other like the bricks of a house wall.

In the reproductive years, the top layer of cells is constantly being

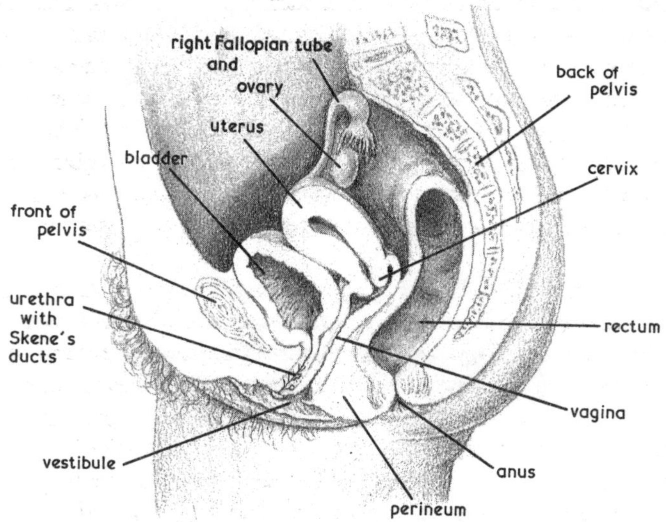

Fig. 3/3 The internal sex organs of a woman

shed into the vagina, where the cells are acted upon by a small bacillus which normally lives there, to produce lactic acid. The lactic acid then kills any contaminating germs that may happen to get into the vagina. Because of this, 'cleansing' vaginal douches, so popular at one time in the USA, are unnecessary. In childhood, the wall of the vagina is thin, and the production of lactic acid does not take place. This is of little importance, however, because the vagina is not usually contaminated at this age. In old age, the lining becomes thin once again, and few cells are shed. Because of this, little or no lactic acid is formed and contaminating germs may grow. This sometimes results in inflammation of the vagina.

The uterus is an even more remarkable organ than the vagina. Before pregnancy it is pear shaped, averages 9cm (3¾in) in length, 6cm (2½in) in width at its widest point, and weighs 60g (2oz). In pregnancy, it enlarges to weigh 1000g (2¼lb), and is able to contain a baby measuring 40cm (17in) in length. It is able to undergo these changes because of the complex structure of its muscle and its exceptional response to the female sex hormones. The uterus is a

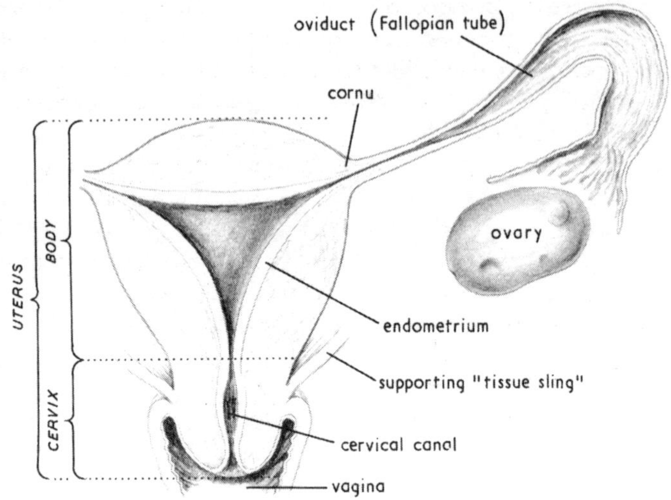

Fig. 3/4 The cavity of the uterus (viewed from the front)

hollow, muscular organ, which is located in the middle of the bony pelvis, lying between the bladder in front and the bowel behind (Fig. 3/4). It is pear shaped, and its muscular front and back walls bulge into the cavity which is normally narrow and slit like, until pregnancy occurs.

Viewed from in front, the cavity is triangular, and is lined with a special tissue made up of glands in a network of cells. This tissue is called the endometrium, and it undergoes changes during each menstrual cycle. For descriptive purposes the uterus is divided into an upper part, or body, and a lower portion, or cervix uteri. The word cervix means neck so that 'cervix uteri' means the neck of the womb. The cavity is narrow in the cervix, where it is called the cervical canal; widest in the body of the uterus; and then narrows again towards the cornu (or horn), where the cavity is continuous with the hollow of the Fallopian tube (Fig. 3/4). The cervix projects into the upper part of the vagina, and is a particular place where cancer sometimes develops.

It is also often infected by sexually transmitted diseases. The ulcer, which forms after infection by syphilis, may occur in the cervix, where it is invisible. Since it is also painless, the woman may not know that she has been infected. This has two dangers. First, she doesn't obtain treatment and has the risk of developing, years later, the serious, disabling third-stage complications of syphilis; and second, she may infect her next sexual partner.

The canal of the cervix is lined with a delicate membrane similar to that of the urethra and Bartholin's gland. It will probably be infected by the germs that cause non-gonococcal genital infections (NGGI) and gonorrhoea if the woman has sex with an infected man. Often the infection causes no symptoms, but may spread from the cervix causing infection of the internal genital organs or may infect the woman's next sexual partner.

Normally the uterus lies bent forward at an angle of 90 degrees to the vagina, resting on the bladder. As the bladder fills, it rotates backwards; as it empties, the uterus falls forward. In about 10 per cent of women the uterus lies bent backwards. This is called retroversion. In the past it was considered a serious condition, causing backache, sterility and many other complaints. There were many operations for its cure. Today it is known that in most cases a retroverted uterus is of no consequence and is not the cause of the symptoms that were attributed to it in the past. However, if NGGI or gonorrhoea spreads upwards through the uterus it may cause pelvic infection and a painful retroverted uterus.

The oviducts (or Fallopian tubes) are two small, hollow tubes, one on each side, which stretch for about 10cm (4in) from the upper part of the uterus to lie in contact with the ovary on each side. The outer end of each oviduct is divided into long finger-like processes, and these are thought to sweep up the egg when it is expelled from the ovary. The oviduct is lined with cells shaped like goblets, which lie between cells with frond-like borders. The oviduct is of great importance, as it is within it that fertilization of the egg takes place, and its secretions probably help to nourish the fertilized egg as it is moved by the cells with long fronds towards the uterus. One of the complications of gonorrhoea is that the infection can spread into the oviducts, which become inflamed and may be damaged, so that the egg is prevented from being fertilized, and the woman is made permanently sterile.

The two ovaries are ovoid-shaped organs, averaging 3.5cm (1½in) in length and 2cm (¾in) in breadth. In the infant they are small, delicate, thin structures, but after puberty they enlarge to reach the adult proportions mentioned. After the menopause, they become small and wrinkled, and in old age are less than half their adult size. Each ovary has a centre made up of small cells and a mesh of blood vessels. Surrounding this is the ovary proper – the cortex – which contains about 200 000 egg cells lying in a cellular bed (the stroma) and outside, again protecting the egg cells and the ovarian stroma, is a thickened layer of tissue. The ovaries are the equivalent of the male testes, and in addition to containing the egg cells on which all human life depends, are a hormone factory producing the female sex hormones, which are so important.

As can be appreciated, the passage within the genital tract extends from the vestibule, along the vagina, through the cervix and uterus, and along the tubes to the ovaries. It is because of this that the male spermatozoa can reach the female egg for fertilization to take place within the oviduct. It also permits infection to spread from the vagina to the ovaries and beyond to cause peritonitis.

Man

In sexual intercourse, the man inserts his erect penis into the woman's vagina, and with a thrusting movement reaches orgasm and ejaculation. If he is a good, considerate lover, he will also seek to help his partner reach orgasm. But if she (or he) inconsiderately has a sexually transmitted disease, his penis is likely to be infected during sexual intercourse.

The external genitals of a man consist of his penis, and his two testes, which lie in the scrotum between his legs, below the root of his penis.

Normally the penis is flaccid and hangs down slackly (Fig. 3/5). In the average adult male it measures 6–14cm (2½–6in) in length but, as in every human characteristic, there is a wide range of normality. When aroused sexually or by direct stimulation, the penis becomes full of blood, stiff, thicker, and points erectly upwards. When this occurs a small penis undergoes a greater increase in size than does a large penis, so that the difference in size between erect penises is not great (Fig. 3/6).

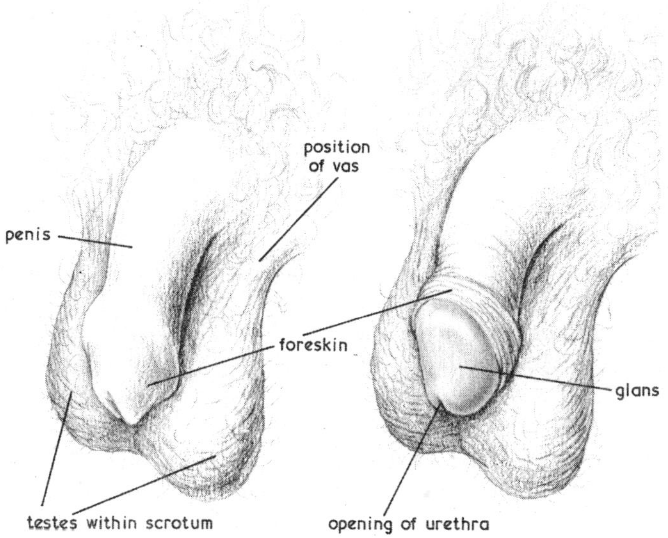

Fig. 3/5 The uncircumcised penis and scrotum. *Right*: the foreskin retracted

If a man has not been circumcised, his foreskin peels back slightly, when his penis is erect, to expose the tip of the underlying head of the penis, which is called the glans penis. The glans is covered with a delicate mucous membrane (similar to that of the mouth) which is richly provided with sensitive nerve receptors. In sexual intercourse, the foreskin peels back so that the entire glans penis is exposed to stimulation as the man thrusts forwards and backwards with his penis in the woman's vagina. Orgasm and ejaculation occur because the glans and shaft of the penis are stimulated by the touch of the vagina in sexual intercourse, or by the hand in masturbation.

The foreskin is prevented from peeling back completely by a band of tissue on the under-surface of the glans, called the frenulum. This band of tissue starts just below the opening of the urethra, which is also called the 'eye' of the penis, and runs back in a small cleft in the glans. The frenulum is also extremely sensitive to touch.

Circumcision, or removal of the foreskin, is done in certain races and in certain religions. The Jews circumcise their boys on the

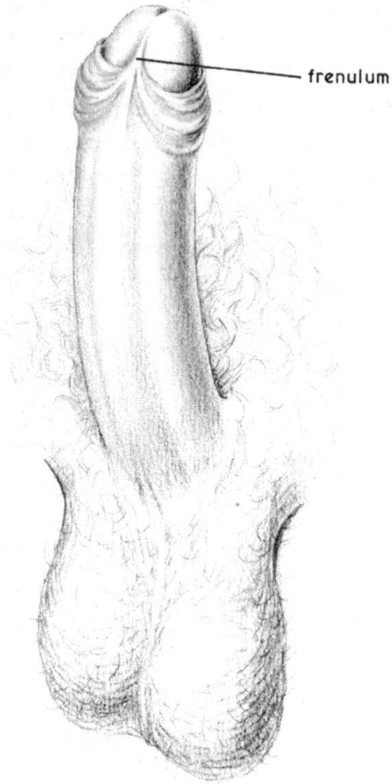

Fig. 3/6 The erect penis showing the glans penis and the frenulum

eighth day of life to fulfil Abraham's covenant with God; the Muslims circumcise their boys at puberty as a symbol of reaching manhood; Aboriginal tribes in the Australian desert circumcise their boys, partly ceremonially as an initiation to manhood, partly for hygiene as the desert sand can irritate the foreskin.

Circumcision of males has a long religious tradition; but in modern times, in some countries and in some social groups it has become a routine performance, not for religious reasons, but because it is the custom. It is said that mothers demand it, doctors profit by it, and babies cannot complain about it. The reasons given are that removal of the foreskin makes the penis cleaner, prevents masturbation, makes it less sensitive so that ejaculation is delayed in coitus, prevents cancer of the cervix in women, and prevents cancer of the penis in men.

The evidence for all these arguments, except the last, is very shaky. The normal foreskin is adherent to the glans of the penis until the infant is at least a year old. After this time it can be drawn back, and if the boy is taught to do this, he can keep his foreskin clean. It will not fix his mind on sex. Nor does the absence of a foreskin prevent masturbation, which is a normal activity. Circumcision does not improve a man's sexual performance, nor does it decrease it: it has no effect. There is no evidence at all that secretions which may be found under the foreskin cause cancer of the cervix in women, although many researchers have tried to prove this. The only men who develop cancer of the foreskin are those who are unhygienic. If, when children, they have been taught to draw back the foreskin and to clean it, cancer will not occur.

None of the so-called medical reasons for circumcision is valid, and there is strong evidence that the foreskin protects the glans of the penis, which is a delicate, sensitive structure.

The organisms causing syphilis usually gain entry to the body of a man through tiny, invisible abrasions in the foreskin, or the skin covering the penis, or through abrasions in the delicate membrane which covers the glans penis, or the frenulum. At the site of infection an ulcer develops.

In the male the urethra is much longer than in the female, measuring about 18cm (8in). It is 'S-shaped' and extends along the under-surface of the penis, through the prostate gland to reach the bladder. Along its course small side tunnels run into small glands. These are called Skene's ducts, and are identical with the Skene's ducts which enter a woman's urethra. And, as in women, the urethra and its accessory glands are lined with a single layer of delicate membrane, through which the gonococcus and chlamydia can easily penetrate (Fig. 3/7).

The gonococcal infection may spread along the urethra and gain entry to the prostate gland which lies just below the bladder. The prostate gland is shaped like a chestnut, and has about 30 tiny ducts which join the urethra, and from which secretions of the prostate enter the urethra. Just behind the prostate, one on each side, are the seminal vesicles. The seminal vesicle is a blind pouch, which develops from each vas deferens. This is a tube which stretches from each testis to the urethra, and along which the sperms pass. The

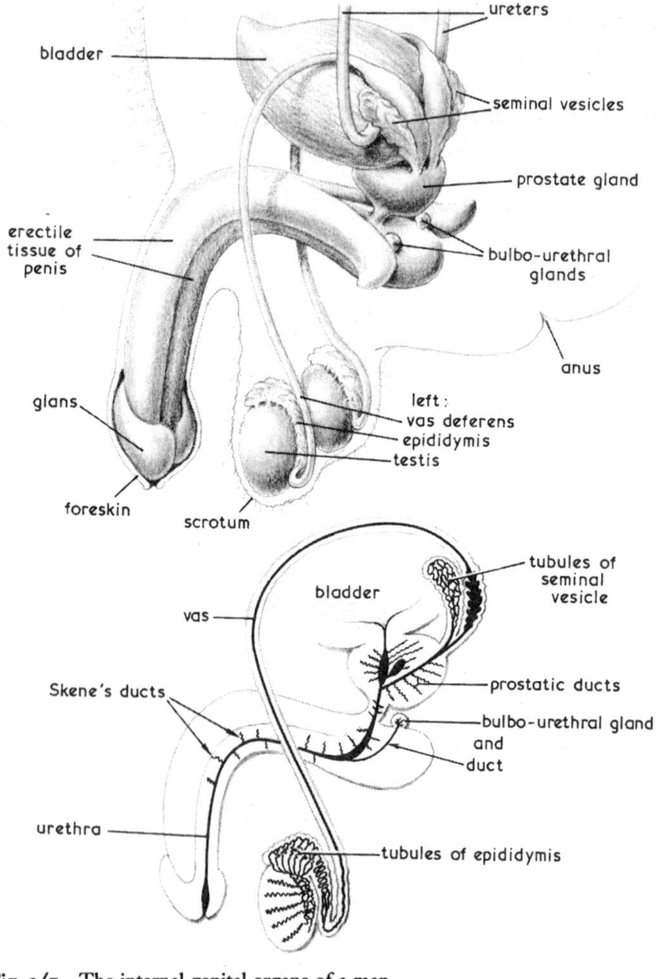

Fig. 3/7 The internal genital organs of a man

seminal vesicles are so called because it was believed that they stored semen, although now it is known that they only store the sticky fluid which forms most of the ejaculate and which nourishes the spermatozoa.

As I mentioned, the two vas deferens stretch from the testes to the urethra. For the first quarter of their length they are outside the body in the scrotum. If you grasp the scrotum where it joins the body and with the thumb in front and the forefinger behind roll the tissues, you will feel a cord-like structure. This is the vas deferens.

As well as permitting the sperms to reach the penis, the vas deferens also permits the gonococcus to reach the epididymis and the testes. The epididymis is a long, twisted, narrow tube, like a tangled ball of string in which the sperms mature before they are ejaculated. It lies alongside and is fixed to its testis. It connects with the vas above, and with the narrow tubules which make up most of the testis below (Fig. 3/8). The lining of the epididymis is very delicate and if infected by the gonococcus may become damaged and

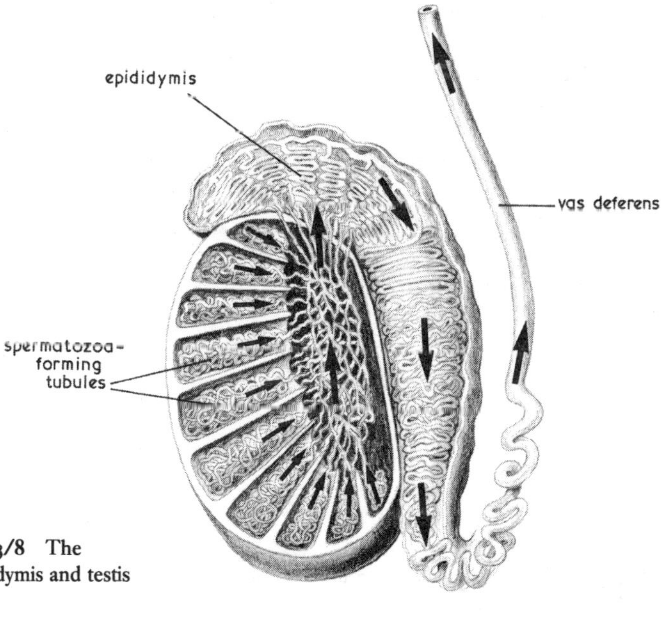

Fig. 3/8 The epididymis and testis

even blocked, which of course makes the man sterile. This is one of the unpleasant complications of untreated gonorrhoea in a man.

The two testes are smooth, oval structures, which are very tender if squeezed, and which lie one in each side of the scrotum. Each testis is made up of about 250 small compartments, like the sections of an orange. Each compartment contains a twisted tube lined by cells. These cells develop and form the spermatozoa from puberty onwards. Between the convolutions of the tubes are special cells which secrete the male hormone testosterone.

It will be appreciated that in the male the genital tract, at least from the prostate onward, is used both by spermatozoa during ejaculation, and by urine during urination. Because of this, infection can spread either to the bladder, or to the testis, with equal ease. This applies particularly to gonococcal infections.

4. About chlamydia infections

In the past 25 years a 'new' sexually transmitted disease has appeared. It is possible that before that date the disease was present but was so mild that medical help was rarely sought. The disease is called non-gonococcal genital infection (NGGI). The dramatic rise in the incidence of NGGI is shown by statistics from several countries. In England and Wales, for example, 11 500 cases were reported from hospital clinics in 1952; 10 years later this had risen to 25 000, by 1972 to over 70 000 and by 1988 the number of cases had risen to 175 000 (Fig. 4/1). This last figure is nearly three times the incidence of gonorrhoeal infections reported in the same year. Similar increases had been reported in other countries.

NGGI affects men and women rather differently, although in

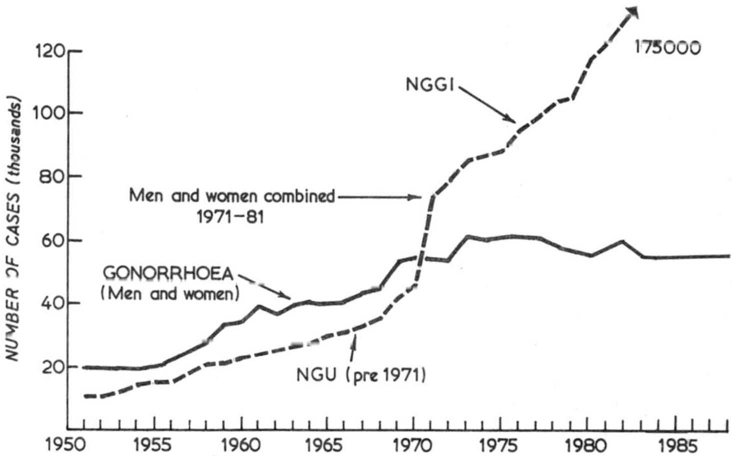

Fig. 4/1 New cases of non-gonococcal genital infection (NGGI) reported in the United Kingdom since 1950

both sexes the most common cause is a tiny organism called *Chlamydia trachomatis*. This organism accounts for over 50 per cent of NGGI in men, and over 80 per cent in women. In men, the urethra is infected, leading to a discharge from the penis. The condition has been given the name non-gonococcal urethritis (NGU). The reason why women do not develop NGU is probably because their urethra is shorter than that of a man and has fewer areas that favour the growth of chlamydia and other organisms. However, chlamydia infects women in a different part of the genital tract. Studies have shown that 30 to 35 per cent of women who have had several sexual partners have symptomless chlamydia infections of the cervix and about 80 per cent of women who have sexual intercourse with an infected man acquire chlamydia infection of the cervix. This 'silent reservoir' is the source of the infection acquired by heterosexual men, and permits NGGI to spread.

It has also become apparent recently that about 20 per cent of men infected with NGU have no symptoms. These men may act as a 'silent reservoir' for the transmission of NGGI. These men have symptomless NGU but may infect their sexual partner, who develops symptoms.

The cervix is also the site where chlamydia infection occurs in women following sexual intercourse with a man who has NGU. Unfortunately, chlamydial infection in women can have disastrous results, causing infection of the internal genital organs. This will be discussed later.

A test has been developed that will identify chlamydial infections of the cells lining the urethra or the cervical canal. A swab is taken by inserting a special cotton wool tipped stick into the woman's cervix or the man's urethra. The swab is rotated through one full circle. The material obtained is placed in a test tube containing a special fluid and sent to a laboratory. It is recommended that the following people are screened for chlamydial infection:

1. Women who have another STD.
2. Women who have evidence of pelvic infection.
3. Women who are suspected or known to have several sexual partners.
4. Heterosexual men who have another STD.

5. Heterosexual men who have casual sex.
6. Heterosexual men who have a recurrence of NGU.
7. Homosexual men with anal symptoms, not due to gonorrhoea or genital herpes.

Recent studies in several Western countries of cervical smears taken from women attending family planning clinics or antenatal clinics show that between 5 and 7 per cent of the smears are infected with chlamydia. The women had no symptoms of infection. There are, as yet, few studies about the prevalence of chlamydia in symptomless men; but as many or more men than women are expected to be infected, as judged by a small investigation of sexually active adolescent men in the USA, when 10 per cent were found to have symptomless urethral infection with chlamydia.

Non-gonococcal genital infection in males

The disease usually starts as an infection of the man's urethra, leading to a discharge from the penis. The appearance of the discharge is identical with that of gonorrhoea and the two sexually transmitted diseases can only be differentiated by examination under a microscope of swabs of the discharge. If the discharge is due to gonorrhoea, the organism causing gonorrhoea will be seen. But if no gonococci are found, the diagnosis is probably non-gonococcal urethritis (NGU).

THE SYMPTOMS OF NGU

Between 7 and 14 days (occasionally longer) after sexual intercourse, usually with a casual partner, the man discovers he has a discharge from his urethra, which may be clear, milky or purulent. Often the discharge is only slight. When the man passes urine, its passage along his urethra may cause discomfort or pain, although often this is only mild. Occasionally the symptoms are more severe: the man develops bladder pain and an urgent and frequent need to pass urine.

If he seeks medical examination he should avoid passing urine for at least 2 hours before seeing the doctor. The doctor may massage his penis along the urethra to try to express a bead of pus. If the doctor has a microscope and is used to staining slides, he may smear some of the pus on a slide, stain it and look at the slide through a microscope. In other cases, where no pus is obtained from the man's urethra, the doctor may ask him to bring a specimen of urine obtained when he first urinated in the morning. This specimen is centrifuged and the sediment obtained is placed on a microscope slide and stained. If a specialized laboratory is available the doctor may also take a sample of the pus and put this in a test-tube containing a fluid substance (culture medium), in which bacteria grow easily. The test-tube is sent to a laboratory, a slide is examined and a culture is made for chlamydia. When the slide is examined no gonococci are found in the material, but many pus cells can be seen (Fig. 4/2). The culture for chlamydia may or may not be positive.

It will be appreciated that clinically NGU is identical with gonorrhoea in its early stages. For this reason, and also because untreated NGU may be followed by unpleasant complications, a man who develops painful urination and a urethral discharge should

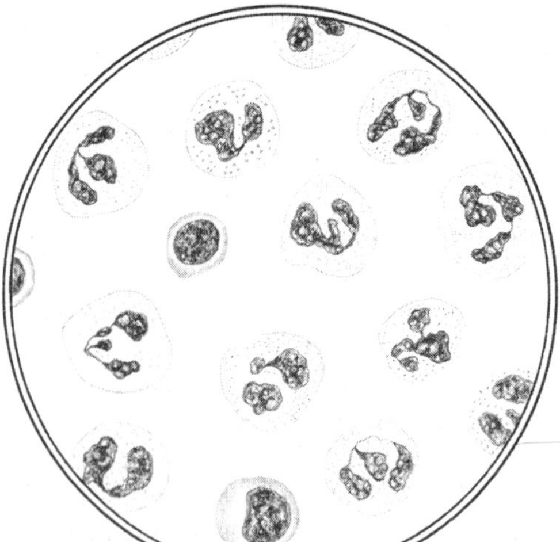

Fig. 4/2 Non-gonococcal urethritis seen through a microscope

seek a medical opinion, and receive appropriate treatment after a diagnosis has been made.

The treatment is simple – to take one of several antibiotics:

1. Doxycycline (Vibramycin); one tablet (100mg) every 12 hours for two doses, then one tablet daily with food or milk for 14 days. The tablet should be swallowed as it may cause irritation of the oesophagus if chewed.
2. Oxytetracycline: two capsules (500mg) 4 times a day for 14 days. The capsule is taken after a meal, during which milk, butter or cheese have not been eaten, as these foods reduce the amount of antibiotic absorbed and the residual amount left in the gut may cause intestinal upset. The cost of oxytetracycline is lower than that of doxycycline.
3. Erythromycin: two capsules (500mg) 4 times a day for 14 days. This antibiotic is chosen for men and women who are sensitive to the tetracyclines (and for women who are pregnant because tetracyline may cause discoloration or damage to the growing teeth of the fetus).
4. Bactrim or Septrin: nine single-strength tablets once each day for 3 days.

During the treatment the person should avoid sexual intercourse and alcohol. The latter seems to increase the resistance to cure.

As a person who has NGU may also have been infected with gonorrhoea, smears and culture are taken at the first visit. The results of the culture usually take 7 days to obtain. It is important that a person who is being treated for NGU should return to the doctor 7 days after starting treatment, and again when treatment is complete, so that further checks can be made. The man's sexual partner, or partners, should also be examined so that chlamydia infection may be detected or excluded.

Complications may occur if the organism causing NGU, usually chlamydia, spreads to the man's bladder or to his prostate gland. If the bladder becomes infected, the man complains of severe pain, especially when he passes urine, which he wants to do all too often, and is often unable to do so because of the pain. If the organism spreads into the prostate gland it causes discomfort deep in the pelvis. Sometimes the spread is without symptoms, but from the warm security of the prostate gland, the disease may affect distant organs.

In fact, a peculiar group of symptoms seems to follow untreated chlamydial urethritis. These are conjunctivitis, urethritis and painful swellings of several of the bigger joints, a form of acute arthritis. The conjunctivitis and urethritis start days, or weeks, after exposure to infection, and settle quite quickly. The arthritis starts rather more slowly and persists. There may be associated fever and a feeling of being vaguely ill. There is reason to believe that the group of symptoms – called a syndrome – is due to an allergic reaction to the persistence of the organism in the body, probably in the prostate gland. It affects between 1 and 3 per cent of men who have had NGU. The syndrome, first described by a Dr Reiter, and subsequently called Reiter's syndrome settles after a few months, and the joints usually recover, but further attacks are usual, and these may lead to permanent damage and deformities of the affected joints.

Many men become affected psychologically. The man becomes depressed, angry and fears that he has another more serious STD, such as AIDS. Some people have persisting or recurrent attacks and laboratory evidence of infection.

Non-gonococcal genital infection in women

NGGI in women are usually without symptoms, at least initially, as the urethra is only occasionally infected. Instead the woman's cervix is infected. It may not spread from here, and the woman's immune defences may eliminate it, but in other cases the infection persists without symptoms, or may spread upwards to infect the woman's genital organs causing pelvic inflammatory disease (PID).

Until recently it was believed that most cases of PID were due to gonorrhoea, but it is now known that most follow an infection by chlamydia, often in association with bacteria that grow in the absence of oxygen (anaerobes). In the past 5 years PID has been diagnosed more frequently in all Western nations. For example, in England and Wales, the reported cases of PID have increased by 70 per cent in the past 15 years (Fig. 4/3). In the USA over 300 000 episodes of PID occur each year and in about 20 per cent the disease leads to permanent damage to the Fallopian tubes. In mild infections the

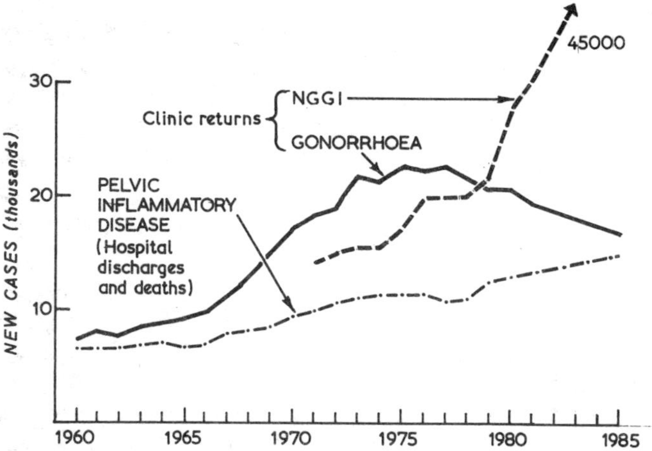

Fig. 4/3 Reported cases of non-gonococcal genital infection, pelvic inflammatory disease and gonorrhoea in women, 1960–88 in England and Wales

damage may not block the tube and will not prevent pregnancy, but if the woman does become pregnant, it is four times as likely for the embryo to lodge in the damaged Fallopian tube.

This is called an ectopic pregnancy. As the placenta invades the wall of the Fallopian tube internal bleeding occurs with severe pain. Surgery is needed to save the woman's life but the embryo is doomed. The incidence of ectopic pregnancy is increasing in all countries. In the USA, the number of ectopic pregnancies has risen from 15 000 in 1965 to over 75 000 in 1989, and in many instances ectopic pregnancy has followed an attack of PID.

If the infection is more severe, the Fallopian tubes are so damaged they become blocked and the sperm and the ovum are unable to meet. The woman is made infertile. Even with new surgical techniques only 15 to 20 per cent of women who have surgery performed on blocked Fallopian tubes, due to infection, will be able to conceive, even if they enter an *in-vitro* fertilization programme.

In severe cases of PID the woman is ill and often has a fever. Her abdomen is painful and tender when examined. If a doctor examines her vaginally, the Fallopian tubes may be felt to be swollen and tender. Not all women present with marked symptoms and often an accurate diagnosis can be made only if the doctor looks at the pelvis through an instrument, like a narrow telescope, called a laparoscope (Fig. 4/4).

If permanent damage to the Fallopian tubes, which makes a woman sterile, is to be avoided, treatment must be given as early as possible. Unfortunately, many women who develop PID have few or no symptoms, and the evidence of the infection is found when the woman fails to become pregnant and is investigated for infertility.

Treatment of diagnosed PID is with the antibiotics prescribed for men who have NGU, usually in combination with a drug called metronidazole, which kills anaerobic bacteria. During treatment the woman should avoid sex and alcohol.

A single attack of NGGI results in damage to the Fallopian tubes

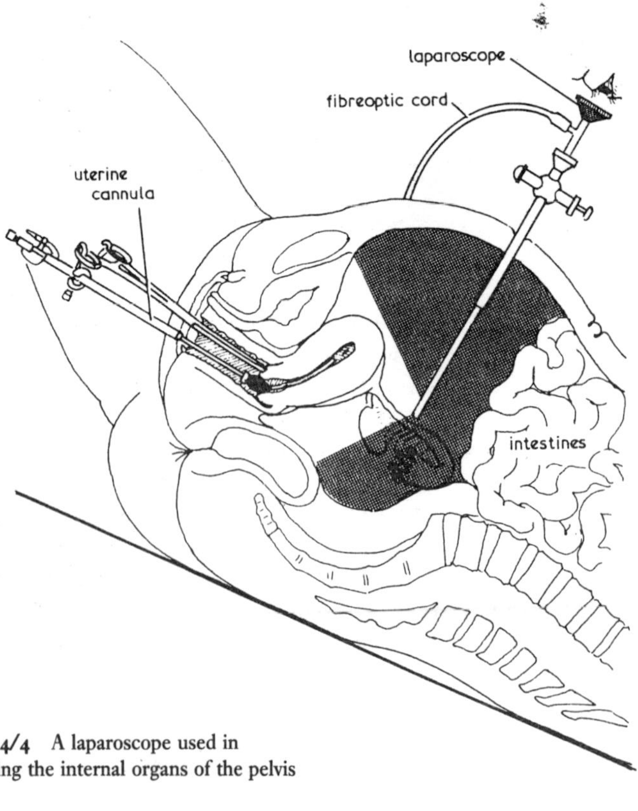

Fig. 4/4 A laparoscope used in viewing the internal organs of the pelvis

in about 12 per cent of cases. If the woman is infected a second time, the percentage of damaged tubes increases to 40 per cent; and after a third attack to 80 per cent. The figures illustrate the dangers of NGGI, and the need for all men who have a urethral discharge to have it investigated. During the period of investigation the man should avoid having sex.

Because of the potentially serious consequences, women who have casual sex with a man whose sexual behaviour is unknown, or who admits to or is suspected of having several sexual partners, should insist that the man wears a condom.

5. About gonorrhoea

As old as recorded history, gonorrhoea has been a by-blow of sexual intercourse. It was mentioned by the Jews in Leviticus, the third book of Moses, and the name of the disease, gonorrhoea, was coined by the ancient Greek physician Galen, in AD 130. The word means 'flow of seed', and the term graphically describes the main feature of the disease.

In most cases, gonorrhoea is spread from person to person by sexual contact and, as its name suggests, the majority of people develop an acute infection of the genito-urinary tract. In some cases, when anal intercourse has taken place, the anal canal may be infected and in other cases the person's throat may be infected with gonorrhoea, if he or she licks or sucks an infected person's genitals. In rare cases gonorrhoea is spread in other ways. One example is the spread of gonorrhoea from an infected mother to the eyes of her infant during childbirth. It is one of the commonest infectious diseases, and it has been estimated that more than 200 million new cases occur each year.

The organism that causes gonorrhoea is a small bean-shaped germ, called *Neisseria gonorrhoeae*, which is transferred during sexual intercourse from the urethra of an infected man to the cervix, the urethra, the throat or the rectum of his female partner, or to the rectum or throat of his male partner, if he is homosexual. It is transferred with equal facility from the urethra, the cervix or the Bartholin's glands of an infected woman to the urethra of an uninfected male partner during sexual intercourse. The urethra, the cervix and the rectum are lined with a single layer of cells, which the gonococcus finds easy to penetrate and, having established a base, it multiplies very quickly. The vagina, which is lined by several layers of cells, is not affected, as the gonococcus is unable to penetrate this 'wall of cells'.

The *Neisseria gonorrhoeae*, or gonococcus, is a very fragile organism, and dies very rapidly if it is not within the warm human body. Small falls in temperature will kill it, and even if the infected discharge from the urethra contaminates clothes or other articles, those articles are rarely infectious, as drying quickly kills the gonococcus. For this reason the story that you can get gonorrhoea from an infected towel, a lavatory seat, or infected clothing, should be remembered for what it is – a story. Very occasionally, a parent or an attendant who has acute gonorrhoea may transfer the germs, by their hands, to the vagina of a young girl, and cause gonorrhoea in the child. This occurs only if the parent first fingers his or her own urethra and then fingers the child's vulva. The wall of the vagina of a girl before she reaches puberty is only one or two cells thick, so that the gonococcus can penetrate it. But it should be stressed that this is a very rare method of catching gonorrhoea, and the most usual method by far is by having sexual intercourse with an infected partner. Gonorrhoea is highly infectious and over 50 per cent of people who have sexual contact with an infected person will acquire the disease.

Gonorrhoea in a man

A man knows he is infected between 3 and 5 days after sexual intercourse. The first thing he notices is that he has developed discomfort or tingling in his urethra. Very quickly a discharge appears, which is creamy, thick and purulent and which drips from his penis (Fig. 5/1). He also finds that it is uncomfortable to pass urine and, when he does, he has a burning feeling in his urethra. The area around the 'eye' of his penis is reddened, but he usually feels quite well apart from the symptoms I have mentioned. If he does not seek treatment, the infection spreads upwards along his urethra and in 10 to 14 days the part of the urethra nearest to his bladder becomes inflamed. When this happens, the burning and pain on passing urine increase, and he may feel unwell, with headaches, or with fever from absorption into his blood of toxic products from the infection. If he still does not seek treatment, the symptoms disappear

Fig. 5/1 Gonorrhoeal urethral discharge

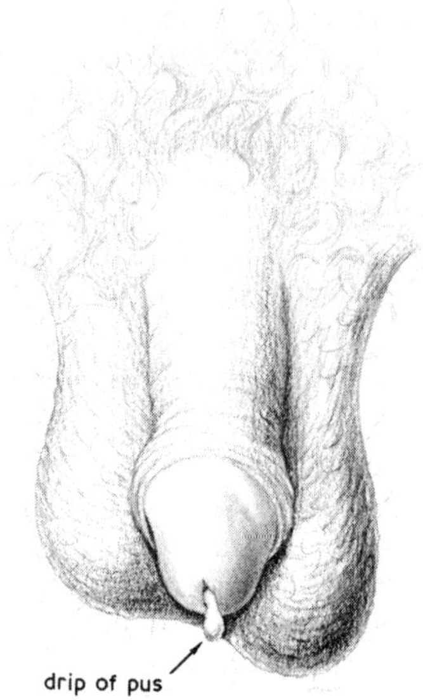

in a few more days, or the disease spreads to affect organs which are adjacent to the urethra, particularly the prostate gland and the bladder, or even to the testis, where it causes an acute inflammation with a painful, swollen testis and the chance of permanent damage which could cause sterility.

It has been reported recently that a small number of men who acquire gonorrhoea have few or no symptoms. Although the proportion of symptomless men is far fewer than that of symptomless women, these men, if promiscuous as most are, will spread the disease.

In the days before antibiotics were available, the only treatment for gonorrhoea was the use of local antiseptics. These were not very efficient and may have aggravated, rather than cured, the disease. In those days, the symptoms of chronic gonorrhoea developed. The most common, and the most painful one, was a narrowing or stricture, of the posterior urethra. This led to difficulty in passing urine, or to the failure to pass urine at all. The treatment was painful, and consisted of pushing narrow metal, or plastic, rods along the urethra to try to stretch the narrowed portion. The operation was called dilatation of the urethral stricture, and the sufferer had to submit to this at frequent intervals.

Gonorrhoea in a woman

In women the pattern of the progress of gonorrhoea is more sinister and more serious. In the first place, between 30 and 50 per cent of infected women have no symptoms, but they can transmit the disease for prolonged periods. They act as a silent reservoir of infection, which considerably complicates the control of gonorrhoea, for a promiscuous woman who has symptomless gonorrhoea can infect a large number of men. Even when women develop symptoms these are usually less marked than in men. This is because a women's urethra is shorter, and is more readily cleansed by passing urine. In fact, one recommended method of avoiding gonorrhoea was to empty the bladder immediately after sexual intercourse. It was not very efficient. The other was for a man to wear a condom when he sought casual sex. This is a more efficient prophylactic method, but may not give complete protection.

If a woman unknowingly harbours the gonococcus or, knowing she has gonorrhoea, fails to have treatment, the disease may spread in several directions within her body. One common, and painful, complication is if one of Bartholin's glands becomes infected. These glands lie deep in the tissues at the entrance of the vulva and supply secretions which make the vagina moist and sexual intercourse more pleasant. If one of the glands becomes infected with gonorrhoea, it becomes swollen, painful and tender.

Occasionally the gonococcus spreads upwards from the cervix, through the uterine cavity, to infect the Fallopian tubes (Fig. 5/2). This seems to occur during menstruation, and if the tubes become infected the woman complains of fever, headache, and pain in her lower abdomen. Examination, particularly pelvic examination, by a doctor causes considerable pain. The sinister sequel of infection of the oviducts, which is termed salpingitis, is that the tubes may become kinked and blocked, causing permanent sterility. If this happens in adolescence, following a chance sexual encounter with an infected male, it may prevent the woman ever having a child.

In both sexes, gonorrhoea may affect the anus and rectum. In

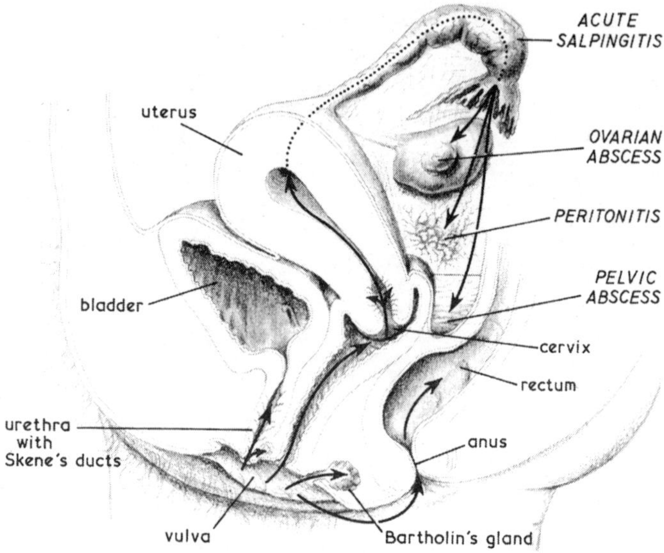

Fig. 5/2 The spread of gonorrhoea in a woman

women this occurs either following anal intercourse by an infected man, or when the infected secretions contaminate the anus during sleep or after defaecation. In males, the infection follows anal intercourse with an infected homosexual partner. In one study made in Denmark, 30 per cent of women with gonorrhoea also had anal infection.

Diagnosis

Gonorrhoea is diagnosed, in the male, by taking a specimen of the urethral discharge and placing it on a slide. After appropriate staining, the slide is examined under a microscope, when clusters of bean-shaped gonococci, which seem to prefer to lie in pairs, are found inside pus cells (Fig. 5/3). In women, the diagnosis is often more difficult and smears are usually taken from the woman's urethra, her upper vagina and her cervix when gonorrhoea is suspected. These smears are placed on special glass dishes which contain a nutrient material and the dishes are heated, or incubated,

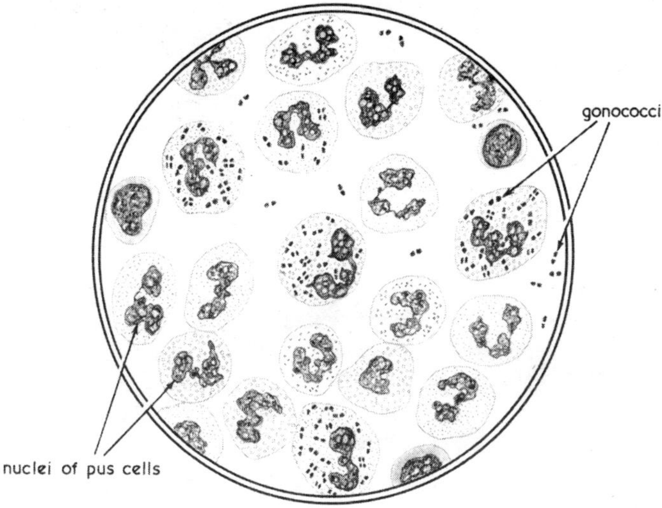

Fig. 5/3 The gonococcus seen through a microscope

for 2 days. In this way any gonococci present will grow and the growth will be seen on the material in the dish. If a specimen from this material is now examined under a microscope the typical bean-shaped germs of gonorrhoea can be identified.

Once the diagnosis has been made, the patient is told by the doctor that he (or she) has gonorrhoea and his help is sought in contacting the sexual partner who gave him the disease. Until the disease is cured the patient must avoid alcohol, as this seems to encourage the disease to relapse, and must obviously avoid sexual intercourse, for he will certainly infect his next partner. He should wash his hands after passing urine or defaecating, and should wash his genitals each day with soap and water, drying them with a towel which *nobody* else uses.

Treatment

The patient is then given treatment. Today, penicillin is the most efficient killer of gonococci, although increasing numbers are becoming relatively resistant to penicillin, so that increasingly higher doses are needed to cure the disease. The reason for resistance is not clear, but it may be due to the abuse of penicillin, given in inadequate doses for inappropriate, or trivial, disorders over the past 20 years. Another reason, particularly in Asia, is that many prostitutes are given a weekly injection of penicillin, supposedly to protect their clients from getting a sexually transmitted disease. The dose is too low to eliminate gonorrhoea from their bodies, and the surviving germs have developed a resistance to most penicillins. Up to 50 per cent of cases of gonorrhoea occurring in Thailand, the Philippines, Malaysia and Vietnam are caused by the resistant strain of gonococci. By the late 1970s, in many nations, between 20 and 30 per cent of all cases of gonorrhoea were relatively resistant to normal doses of penicillin. It has also become increasingly obvious that the more simple the treatment the more effective it is. This has meant that new strategies have had to be developed.

Penicillin is the most commonly prescribed treatment but medical reserch has discovered that penicillin is more effective in killing resistant gonococci if another drug is given at the same time. The usual method in the treatment of gonorrhoea is for the patient to take two tablets of this drug, called probenecid, at the time of receiving the penicillin, and a further tablet 6 and 12 hours later. Probenecid blocks the excretion of penicillin from the kidneys enabling higher levels to be obtained in the blood. This gives penicillin a more lethal effect on the gonococcus.

In most cases of genital or rectal gonorrhoea, penicillin is given by mouth in tablet form. Currently, amoxycillin is favoured and 3g (i.e. six 500mg capsules) are taken in a single dose, with 1g (2 tablets) of probenecid. Six and 12 hours later a further tablet of probenecid is taken. If gonorrhoea has infected the throat, amoxycillin and probenecid are given for 3 days in a smaller dose. An alternative to amoxycillin is to give doxycycline (Vibramycin) 200mg (2 tablets) on diagnosis and 100mg twice a day for 6 days.

If the gonorrhoea has spread and has caused infection in the pelvis of a woman, or the testes of a man, larger doses of amoxycillin are given for a longer period of time. For penicillin-resistant gonorrhoea, which was first diagnosed in South-east Asia and today is the cause of 10–25 per cent of cases in many western countries, other antibiotics are preferred. These are ceftriaxone and spectinomycin, which are given as a single injection into the muscles of the buttock. In most cases the antibiotic cures the patient, but since gonorrhoea may lurk in the body it is essential that every patient re-attends the doctor or the hospital clinic for follow-up. 7 days after receiving the penicillin the patient passes a specimen of urine which is examined by the doctor, who also takes further smears from the urethra (and from the cervix if the patient is a woman). In the case of homosexual men, specimens are taken from the rectum for examination. The smears are examined under a microscope and 'cultured' to make sure that no gonococci are still present.

Because at least 25 per cent of people infected with gonorrhoea are infected at the same time with chlamydia, many doctors now give a course of doxycycline (see page 49) immediately after the person has taken the amoxycillin. Other doctors recommend that amoxycillin and doxycycline are replaced by a drug called trimethoprim-sulphamethoxazole (co-trimoxazole). This drug is more widely known by its trade names of Bactrim and Septrin. Nine single-strength tablets of Bactrim or Septrin are taken once each day for 3 days. This drug regimen seems more effective than the other drugs in eliminating chlamydia as well as gonococci.

As discussed in Chapter 4, chlamydia (and other organisms) causes NGU in men and NGGI in women. An infected man who has not been cured by the treatment for gonorrhoea will develop a urethral discharge 5 to 25 days after receiving treatment, but an infected woman usually has no symptoms. As chlamydia is present in her cervix she is likely to infect her next sexual partner.

It is important that a person treated for gonorrhoea returns to see the doctor 10 days after completing treatment for a check-up. A man is considered cured if he has no discharge from his urethra and a specimen of his urine is clear. If a discharge from the urethra persists, a further smear is made and examined under a microscope. If gonococci are seen on a stained slide, a culture is sent to the laboratory to check if it is one of the penicillin-resistant strains. If no gonococci are seen, the man is treated for NGU (see page 47). During the course of treatment the doctor also makes tests to determine whether the patient has been infected with syphilis at the same time he or she acquired gonorrhoea. This is important as the dose of antibiotics given to cure gonorrhoea is insufficient to cure syphilis. If syphilis is detected, the patient is given a further course of penicillin.

Because gonorrhoea is 'silent' in so many women, and because of its unpleasant consequences both to the woman herself and her sexual partners, an even more careful follow-up has to be made after a woman has been treated for gonorrhoea. She needs to be examined 5 to 7 days after completing treatment when smears are taken from her urethra, her vagina and her cervix. These are repeated in the first days after her next menstrual period. If the tests are negative at each examination a woman can be sure that she has been cured of gonorrhoea.

6. About genital warts

Genital warts, which occur on the penis, on the vulva or around the anus have been known and written about since the days of ancient Greece. The warts may be single or may be multiple, covering large areas of the skin and, in the case of women, extending into the vagina. They occur only after sexual maturity has been reached, and they have a peak age incidence between the ages of 25 and 35 in men and women. They are four times as common as genital herpes, about 6 per cent of people being infected. This is also the peak age incidence of gonorrhoea, which suggests that they are spread by sexual intercourse. In men the foreskin, the frenulum, and the lower edge of the glans penis are most frequently affected (Fig. 6/1), while in women the warts are most frequently found on the area around the vaginal entrance and the inner surface of the labia majora (Fig. 6/2), but any part of the vulva, vagina or the cervix may be affected. It is only recently that the infection of the cervix has been recognized, but the consequences of this infection may be serious.

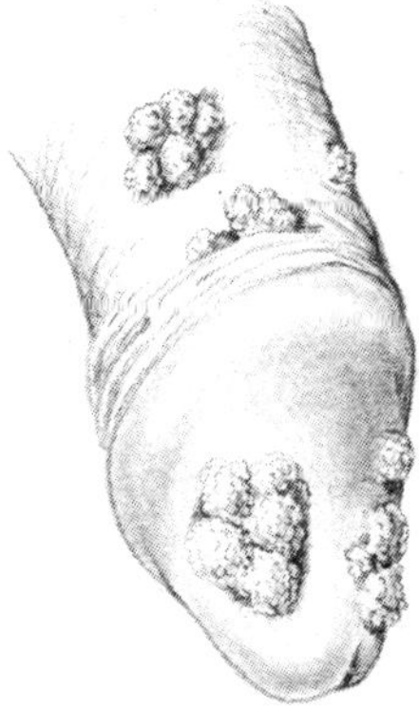

Fig. 6/1 Severe genital warts on the penis; in many cases the warts are invisible

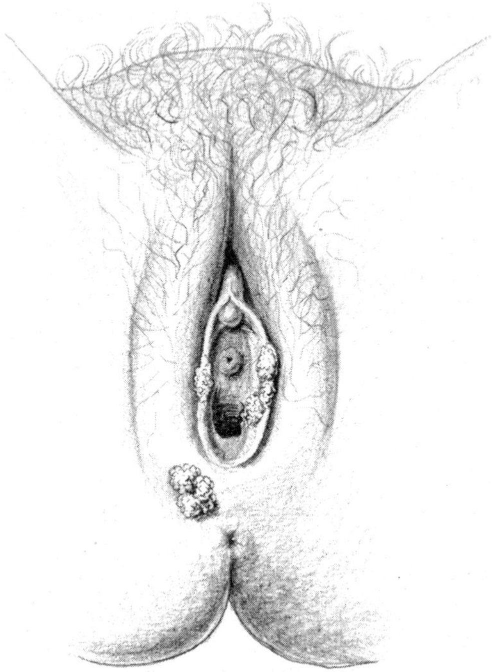

Fig. 6/2 Genital warts on the vulva

Genital warts arise from infection by one or more of the human papilloma viruses (HPV). This family of viruses is common and is the cause of warts on various parts of the body. Warts that appear on the genital areas of men and women are usually due to the stains of the virus numbered 6, 16 or 18. The wart virus enters the skin of the vulva or the penis, or the tissues (mucous membrane) of the penis or urethra, or those of the vagina or the cervix during sexual intercourse with an infected partner. The virus tends to remain quiet and warts only develop after about 3 months. The warts may be obvious or may only be detected by looking at the man's penis or at the woman's vagina or cervix using a magnifying glass. Once they have appeared they tend to spread.

The warts may spread to the area around the anus, but if they are only found in this area, it is suggestive that anal sexual intercourse has taken place. In a study of 60 men and 8 women who had anal warts, Dr Oriel of London found that 83 per cent of the men and 62 per cent of the women said that they practised anal intercourse.

Until recently it was believed that apart from looking unsightly, genital warts were harmless. It is now known that this is untrue. The wart virus may enter and live in the cells which cover the cervix or the vagina, and may alter the cells so that they may become cancerous. This event is most likely to occur in the cells that cover the cervix. Fortunately the abnormal cells can be detected long before cancer develops if women who are sexually active have regular checks. At this check-up a sample of the cells covering the cervix is removed by gently scraping the cervix with a wooden or plastic stick or a small specially designed brush. This is the Pap smear. If abnormal cells are detected many doctors believe that the cervix should be inspected with an instrument called a colposcope which magnifies the cervix and enables abnormalities invisible to the eye to be detected and treated.

Warts detected on the vulva or around the anus, which are not too extensive, are painted by a health professional with a substance called podophyllin, which seeps into the wart and kills the virus. Podophyllin is carefully applied to each wart, making sure that the surrounding skin is not touched, as the substance burns. The 'paint' is allowed to dry. The patient then goes home, and 2 hours later washes the area with soap and water to remove any traces of podophyllin which have not been absorbed into the wart.

In most cases the paint has to be reapplied each week for 3 or 4 weeks. The warts shrivel and drop off as the infected cells die, leaving a clear skin.

Recently a derivative of podophyllin called podophyllotoxin or podofilox has been developed, which the infected person can apply to the warts himself or herself. The person applies the substance to the genital warts twice a day for 3 days, taking care to avoid putting it on adjacent unaffected skin. After a 4-day interval the treatment is repeated. This eliminates the warts in about 80 per cent of cases.

One person in every five who applies podophyllin or podofilox has some degree of a burning feeling or itching, which lasts for a day or two.

Unfortunately, the genital warts recur at the same or a different place in one third of people infected.

When the warts are extensive or infect the penis, the vagina or the cervix, they are treated by burning them with an electric cautery or vaporizing them with a laser. Burning is more painful than laser treatment and is usually done after the woman has been given a general anaesthetic. Laser treatment may be done under local anaesthesia or a general anaesthetic.

Following treatment the treated area (which may include skin surrounding the wart) requires 3 to 6 weeks to heal. During this time, ointments may be applied which will reduce the discomfort; and intercourse should be avoided.

Because of the potential dangers of infection by the genital wart virus, particularly to women, if the sexual behaviour of the partner is unknown, a condom should be used as a protection during sexual intercourse. Very small warts on a man's penis which are invisible to the naked eye, may be detected if he wraps a cloth soaked in vinegar around it, and leaves it there for 5 minutes. If small white patches are observed on the penis when the cloth is removed, wart virus infection may be suspected. In this case the man should visit a doctor who will look at the man's penis with a magnifying glass to determine if there are any warts. In men the virus usually dies after a few weeks, because the skin and glans of the penis tends to be dry, so that additional treatment may be unnecessary. But some doctors believe that to prevent any possibility of further transmission, the man should be treated. Trichloracetic acid is applied to each white area with a swab stick. This may cause a temporary burning sensation. After 30–60 seconds the man washes his genitals to remove any excess trichloracetic acid. Treatment may need to be repeated after 2–3 weeks, and the man should use a condom during sexual intercourse until the lesions have gone.

A problem in leaving warts untreated in women is that the virus which causes them *may* be a factor in the development of cancer of the uterine cervix 10 or more years later. Because of this possibility and the problem of treating vaginal warts, a new treatment using interferon cream is being investigated. Interferon is produced from white blood cells, specifically attacks viruses, and is extremely expensive. However, in selected cases of warts it may be the answer.

7. About genital herpes

In the past 10 years, genital herpes has been diagnosed by doctors with increasing frequency. In the USA, for example, at least 300 000 new cases are diagnosed each year compared with one-tenth the number 10 years ago.

The actual number of people infected with the herpes virus is unknown. Risk of infection depends on the person's sexual behaviours. For example, a study in the USA showed that 80 per cent of prostitutes, and about 25 per cent of healthy adults had antibodies to the genital herpes virus in their blood, indicating that they had been infected at some time. However, a much smaller number of people have active infection and are potentially infectious to others during sexual intercourse. It is also true that a small number of people who have no active infection may still shed the virus and infect a sexual partner.

It is not clear why there has been an increase in the number of people being diagnosed as having genital herpes, but the increase led in the early 1980s to a number of emotive articles in magazines and newspapers about genital herpes, which produced a hysterical reaction among many people. The articles and programmes may have been intended to inform and to help the community understand more about the new epidemic. They may have been written or produced to sell the medium in which they appeared, because they dealt with a disease spread by sexual contact, for which there was no cure, and which might be considered as the revenge of a wrathful deity on those who enjoyed 'casual sex'.

The reality is that genital herpes is a very old disease. It is caused by a virus. Herpes viruses have probably infected mankind for at least 2 million years. In fact, blood tests to detect if a person has had herpes reveal that over half of all adults have been infected with the

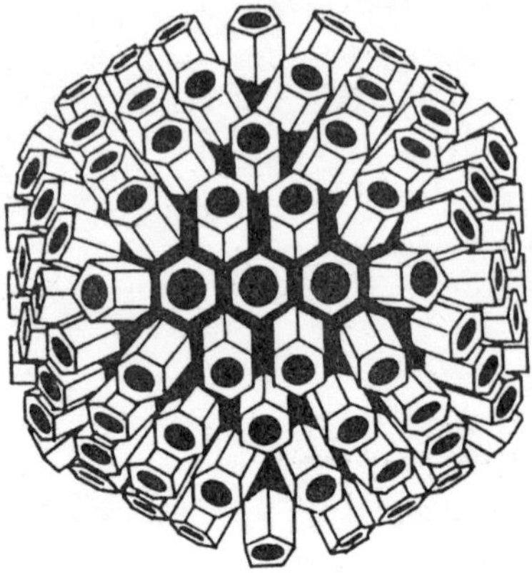

Fig. 7/1 The herpes virus 'shell' or 'capsid'

genital herpes virus (herpes simplex virus, type 2 (HSV 2)), but in most cases the infection was unnoticed.

The herpes virus is a tiny organism composed of a core of coiled, double-stranded nucleic acid (DNA) surrounded by a honeycomb-like covering of protein, and outside that a loose envelope of a fatty substance (Fig. 7/1).

Viruses are so small that one thousand of them would fit into the width of a red blood cell; and 300 red blood cells would fit across the point of a pin. Viruses are inert unless they enter a living cell when they 'reprogram' the cell to produce multiple copies of the invading virus. The virus does this by a process of fusion: the DNA core of the virus enters the nucleus of the infected cell and fuses with the DNA of the nucleus. The nucleus then commands the cell to produce viral DNA and the protein covering. If these are covered with the fatty envelope they become active viral particles. As the viral particles multiply the cell is killed and virus is shed into the body or on to its surface (Fig. 7/2) where it is inert until it enters another living cell, or is killed by sunshine.

The herpes virus does not differ in its appearance from other viruses but has specific characteristics which have enabled scientists to identify it. About 50 herpes viruses which infect mammals have been identified, but only five are known to infect man. These are the two viruses that cause glandular fever (infectious mononucleosis), the Epstein-Barr virus and the cytomegalovirus; one virus, the

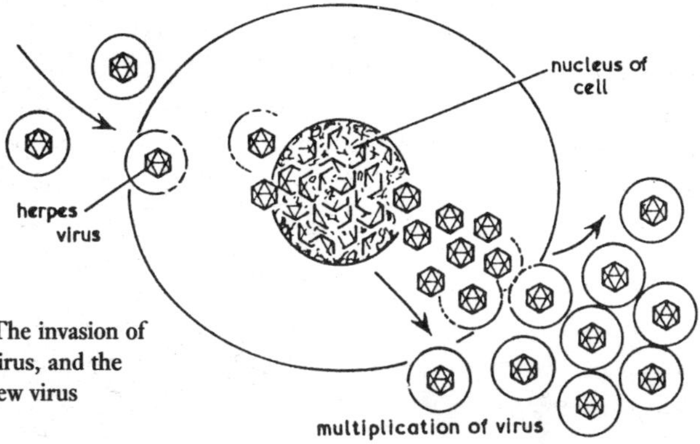

Fig. 7/2 The invasion of a cell by a virus, and the release of new virus particles

varicella virus, which causes chicken-pox in children, and in later life causes shingles; and the two herpes simplex viruses. The first is the herpes simplex virus which usually causes cold sores (herpes simplex virus, type 1 (HSV 1)); and the second herpes simplex virus usually causes genital ulcers (herpes simplex virus, type 2 (HSV 2)).

Chicken-pox (varicella) virus and HSV viruses behave similarly, while the Epstein-Barr virus and the cytomegalovirus behave in another way. Varicella causes chicken-pox in children. During the illness most of the virus enters the bloodstream where it causes a reaction, inducing the body to make antibodies which circulate in the blood and specifically seek out and kill the virus. Some of the virus shed from the skin blisters does not enter the blood but travels down the nerve that supplies that area of the skin. When it reaches a swollen part of the nerve, called a ganglion, near the spinal cord, it lodges in the ganglion and remains there throughout the person's life, probably being kept in check by the circulating anti-virus antibody (Fig. 7/3).

As the person grows older, the level of circulating antibody may fall. If this coincides with an event, the nature of which is not known at present, the virus may travel back along the nerve, usually to the skin, and produce the crop of painful blisters that is called shingles. The blistered cells of the skin produce virus, and this may infect a nurse or doctor who is caring for the person who has shingles. Herpes simplex virus operates similarly. The other two herpes

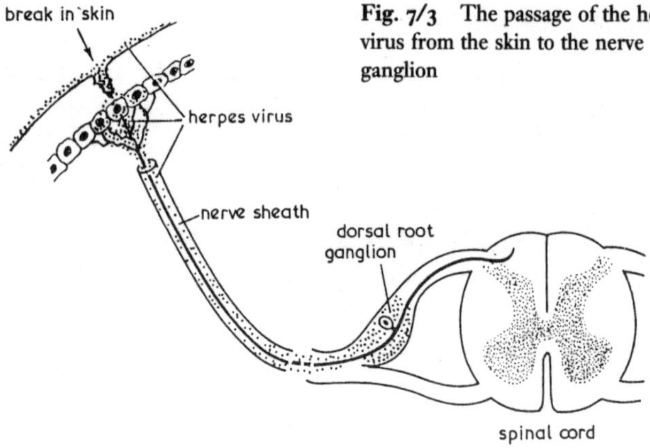

Fig. 7/3 The passage of the herpes virus from the skin to the nerve ganglion

viruses, which cause glandular fever, do not invade nerves but live in white blood cells. Nearly every person has been infected with the glandular fever viruses but only a very few become ill. In most the infection is symptomless.

This is also true of herpes simplex virus type 1 (HSV 1). By the time most people reach adulthood they have been infected by HSV 1 and have developed antibodies against the virus in their blood, although only a few have had cold sores on their lips or nose.

In contrast, fewer people have been infected with HSV 2 during childhood or early adolescence as the virus is usually spread by sexual contact. This is shown by the fact that up to 90 per cent of prostitutes have antibodies to HSV 2 in their blood compared with less than 3 per cent of nuns. This finding led to the belief that HSV 1 infected *only* the lips and HSV 2 infected *only* the genitals. This belief is now known to be false, and the change may be due to the increase in oral sex. Today both HSV 1 and HSV 2 may cause genital herpes, although most infections are due to HSV 2. About half of the people infected with HSV 2 will have no symptoms, at least as judged by the fact that 30 to 60 per cent of adults have antibodies to HSV 2 in their blood, and deny they have had blisters on their genitals. The remainder develop symptoms when they are infected with genital herpes.

Initial attack of genital herpes

The first attack of genital herpes is the worst. The attack usually follows sexual contact with another person who at the time was recovering from an attack of herpes. The sexual contact may be genital, oral or anal.

In 85 per cent of cases the first attack is due to infection with HSV 2; and in 15 per cent the infection is caused by HSV 1. Between 5 and 7 days after the sexual contact, a man develops a small itchy area on the shaft of his penis (Fig. 7/4), and a woman a similar itchy area on the inner surface of her labia majora. In a few people, headache and fever may occur. In others, the person will feel 'off colour' and think that he or she may be developing influenza.

Within 24 hours of the development of the symptoms, small crops of painful, reddish bumps appear in the itchy area, and by the next day have become small blisters. The area is very tender and painful.

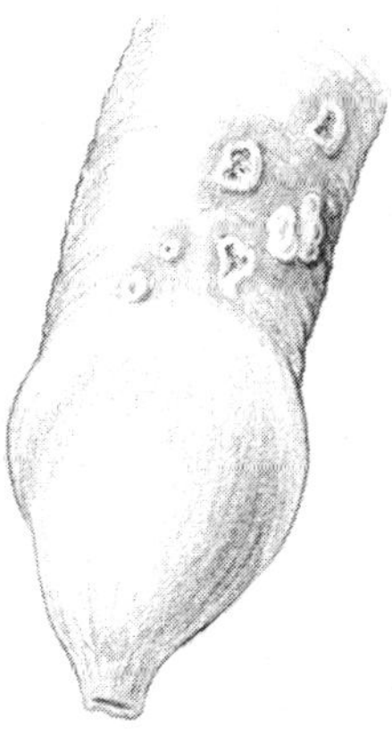

Fig. 7/4 Genital herpes in a man

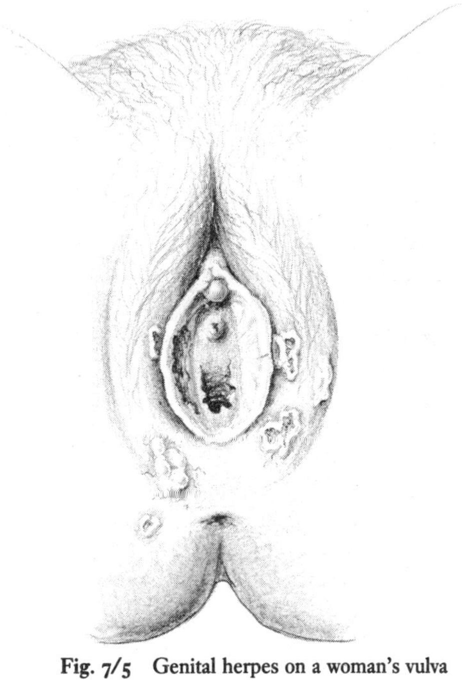

Fig. 7/5 Genital herpes on a woman's vulva

Sometimes the labia become so swollen that urination is difficult and painful. The fluid in the blisters is clear and if a sample is taken and looked at through an electron microscope, or added to a tissue culture, herpes virus particles can be seen. The fluid soon becomes yellow and the blisters burst, leaving a crop of painful ulcers (Fig. 7/5). Over 4 or 5 days the ulcers crust over and heal slowly, the healing being complete in about 7 to 12 days from the appearance of the first blisters. During this time, and for about 7 days after the attack, the person is shedding virus from the infected area and can pass on herpes if he or she has sexual contact with another person.

During the initial infection the person should wear panties or underpants at night lest inadvertently she or he scratches the blistered areas and transfers the virus to the eyes, which may be serious. As well, after touching the area or applying drugs, the hands should be washed.

Recurrent genital herpes

A recurrence occurs when, for some reason, the herpes virus in the nerve ganglion makes its way along the nerve to the area of the skin or mucous membrane that was infected initially. What triggers the virus to travel is unknown. Some women believe that the reason is a hormonal change, as they report that the attack is related to the menstrual period or occurs during the premenstrual week, but other studies have shown no such relationship. 'Stress' or a change in personal relationships has been implicated. Once again, careful investigation has failed to establish either of these problems as a cause, although one British study by two psychiatrists found that people showing hidden psychiatric illness (as estimated by a questionnaire, called the General Health Questionnaire) were more likely to develop a recurrence of genital herpes. The recurrences are not due to an increased frequency of sexual intercourse or a change in sexual partners.

Whatever the cause, once the virus gets into the skin it may lie dormant (or perhaps be shed in small amounts) until it is eliminated by the body's defences, or it may provoke a recurrent crop of blisters. It is known that if the blisters occur, the person is infectious to a sexual partner. It is not known if the person who sheds virus, without any clinical signs of herpes, is infectious; the probability is that he or she is not, which should reassure many sufferers from herpes.

Recurrent attacks of genital herpes affect an unknown number of men and women. Some experts claim that 70 per cent of people have recurrent attacks, some claim that 30 per cent have them, some claim that as few as 1 or 2 per cent have them. A problem is that many recurrent attacks are not reported and with the recent hysteria about herpes any small lump on the genitals may be self-diagnosed as herpes although it is not.

One calculation suggests that about 40 per cent of people infected with herpes will have a single further attack, while between 1 and 5 per cent will have repeated attacks of genital herpes, occurring at longer and longer intervals.

The sequence of events in a recurrent attack is the same as that of the initial attack, but the burning–blistering–ulceration–scabbing–healing process occurs more quickly, the whole episode lasting 5 to 10 days, although the virus may be shed for 3 days more. During this period the person can infect a sexual partner. Pain occurs with recurrent genital herpes but is less severe and lasts for a shorter time than with an initial attack.

The interval between recurrences varies considerably; some people have recurrences every 2 months or more frequently; some people every 2 to 6 months, some only once a year or less frequently.

The psychological effects of recurrent genital herpes on a person's sexuality may be considerable. Some men, who have acquired genital herpes from an extra-marital source, develop erectile failure so that they may avoid the possibility of infecting their marital partner. Some women avoid sexual intercourse for the same reason, telling their husbands that intercourse has become too painful. The fear of transmitting herpes to a partner, the anger that the infection may have been acquired from the partner (implying that he or she has been unfaithful) and the guilt that may follow being infected in a casual encounter, may disturb the person's sexual relationship. In turn, the disruption of the sexual relationship may disturb the overall relationship, with resulting marital distress, requiring counselling.

How is herpes diagnosed?

The only sure way of diagnosing genital herpes is to take a swab from the ulcers (and in the case of women, the cervix of the uterus) and to send this in a special transport fluid to a viral laboratory. There the virus is grown in tissue culture. Occasionally virus particles may be identified under an electron microscope in fluid obtained from the blisters; but the method has limitations and it takes from 3 to 10 days to obtain a positive result. Recently a 24-hour test has been developed. A swab from the suspected lesion is placed in culture for 24 hours and then stained with a special stain which fluoresces if the virus is present. This test is particularly useful in late pregnancy.

A test is available to determine whether a person has had HSV 1 or HSV 2 in the past. The test measures the level of anti-herpes antibody in the person's blood. Using this test, it has been found that between 40 and 70 per cent of adults have been infected with HSV 1 (although in most it was symptomless) and 20 to 50 per cent have been infected with HSV 2 (again most were unaware that they had been infected). More people in the poorer classes seem to have HSV antibodies in the blood.

Can genital herpes be transmitted if there are no blisters?

One study of six women, who had swabs taken from their labia and their cervix at weekly intervals for 30 weeks, showed that one woman shed virus from her vulva and one from her cervix on one occasion, and did not develop herpes blisters. However, there is no evidence that a sexual partner will be infected by this chance viral shedding.

Genital herpes in pregnancy

About one woman in every 1000 will acquire genital herpes and an unknown number of women will have a recurrence of genital herpes during pregnancy. Genital herpes does not affect the course of the pregnancy and the baby, snug in the uterus, is unlikely to be infected, except in severe initial infections, and even then only rarely. If infection occurs in the first half of pregnancy it may lead to an abortion (miscarriage) of the infected baby. If the woman is shedding herpes virus from the lesions of her vulva or from her cervix during the birth of the baby, one newborn baby in every two will be infected with herpes.

Two-thirds of the babies who develop herpes at birth die, and about half of the survivors suffer permanent brain or eye damage. The reason for this sinister outcome of a herpes virus infection is that the newborn baby's immunological defence mechanisms are not fully developed, so that the virus easily multiplies in his or her body.

Luckily, symptomless shedding of HSV 2 virus from the cervix or vulva in pregnancy is uncommon. In a study in the USA of over 800 pregnant women, investigated in late pregnancy by taking swabs at intervals (3000 in all), only one swab in every 300 showed herpes virus. However, infection of the baby during childbirth is still a problem. The chance of the baby's being infected is reduced very considerably if women who have an initial infection of genital herpes and women who develop a recurrent attack during pregnancy are 'screened' from 8 weeks before the baby is due to be born. Every week, or second week, a swab is taken from the woman's cervix and sent in a special fluid to a virus laboratory for tissue culture. The result is obtained within 2 to 4 days. A positive culture found at the time labour starts is an indication for a caesarean section so that the baby doesn't have to journey through an area where virus is being shed. If the culture is negative and there are no genital herpes ulcers on the woman's vulva, the baby may be born in the normal way. It has to be stated that the benefit of doing cultures has been questioned recently.

Does genital herpes cause cancer?

Is herpes virus a cause of cancer of the cervix? At present there is no real evidence that it is. After all, large numbers of women have had genital herpes but only a few develop cervical cancer. It is true that some studies show that women with cervical cancer have higher levels of anti-herpes antibodies in their blood than women who do not have cancer, but this does not mean that herpes virus causes cancer. The connection may be that women who have multiple sexual partners are more likely to acquire genital herpes and seem to be more likely to develop cervical cancer later in life. In other words, the lifestyle of the woman may be the link.

A woman who has genital herpes should not panic in the belief she will develop cervical cancer. She is probably not much more likely than any other woman to develop it. But, as a precaution, she should have swabs taken from her cervix (Pap smears) every one or two years and they should be examined for abnormal cells.

The treatment of genital herpes

In spite of much investigation, the trial of many new drugs, and anecdotal reports, until recently no drug was available that specifically cured genital herpes. Most of the drugs used in the past have been applied to the blisters or ulcers (Table 7/1). As the virus tracks

Table 7/1 Previously tried remedies for genital herpes

DRUGS USED TO TREAT GENITAL HERPES – NO EVIDENCE THAT THEY HAVE ANY VALUE	
Zinc	50–100mg daily orally
Vitamin C in megadoses by mouth	
Yoghurt	applied to blisters
Vegemite	applied to blisters
Herbal remedies	applied to blisters
Ether	applied to blisters
DRUGS TRIED AND ABANDONED AS EITHER INEFFECTIVE OR DANGEROUS	
Influenza vaccine	
Painting with a photosensitive (heterocyclic) dye and exposing to fluorescent light	
idoxuridine	(Stoxil)
cytarabine	(Cytosar)
vidarabine	(Vira-A)

down the nerve supplying the area it is most unlikely that genital herpes can be cured by local applications, although the discomfort may be relieved. For this reason the treatment of genital herpes will be considered under two headings: the treatment of the local symptoms, and specific treatment.

LOCAL TREATMENT

Genital herpes, particularly the initial infection causes considerable pain and distress, particularly among women, whose external genitals (vulva) may become swollen and tender. The swelling and the painful ulcers may make urination agonizing, in which case the woman may need to have a tube (catheter) put in her bladder temporarily. Local applications of ice or an analgesic jelly give relief, but only for a short time. Another method of obtaining some relief is to put a few crystals of potassium permanganate in a warm bath and for the woman to sit in it.

The recent development of the antiviral substance, acyclovir, may offer hope. In early trials, acyclovir ointment applied to the blisters every 6 hours reduced the pain, the swelling and the time the virus was shed. The earlier the ointment was applied the better and quicker the relief. Unfortunately, benefits are found only in primary infections, and acyclovir ointment does not seem very effective in recurrent attacks.

SPECIFIC TREATMENT

Acyclovir is the only drug which has been shown to have any real effect in reducing the severity of the symptoms of initial lesions, making healing more rapid and reducing considerably the time that virus is shed. Acyclovir may be given by intravenous injection, or by mouth, which seems as effective.

Acyclovir given at the time symptoms start does not seem to make much difference to the duration of, or the discomfort associated with, recurrent herpes. Recent research in Britain and the USA, has found that if acyclovir is given prophylactically (that is when there are no symptoms), in a dose of 200mg 2 to 4 times a day, the frequency of attacks of recurrent genital herpes is reduced considerably.

However, the drug is expensive (1 year's supply costing over $1500 (£1000)), and the possible side-effects of long-term use are unknown. Because of this it should only be used, at present, for people who have at least one recurrent attack every month.

According to an American expert 'acyclovir is a first-generation anti-viral agent, not a cure'. Research scientists are working on second-generation anti-viral drugs which may prove more effective.

Other drugs used in the past (Table 7/1) have not been shown to provide any real benefit compared with placebo. However, if a person who has genital herpes *believes* that one of them helps, he or she should not be dissuaded from using the drug, or the vitamin he chooses.

The psychological effects of having herpes

It is neither sensible nor helpful to consider genital herpes as incurable. There are many viruses that stay in our bodies for life. Most do not cause further infections and this applies to the herpes virus. If your approach to herpes is positive it will become a relatively insignificant part of your life. Those people who have recurrent herpes have no way of predicting if and when a further attack will occur. For most people the number of recurrences depends on how fit you are, both physically and emotionally. A recurrence is more likely if you are under stress or are run down. Some women develop a recurrence in the week before menstruation, some men and women have a recurrence if they work too many hours, drink too much alcohol, do not get enough sleep or eat a poor diet.

A positive approach to your life and to genital herpes is important. If you have recurrent herpes do not blame yourself, or your partner. You may have had the first infection long ago and it was so mild that you did not know you had it. Accept that you have recurrent herpes, and avoid those actions that seem to bring on attacks. Do not let the genital herpes affect your relationships, or reduce your desire for intimacy.

If you find that the trauma of having recurrent genital herpes is affecting your life, seek help and talk to a counsellor, who may be a doctor or a psychologist. Remember, too, that acyclovir in a dose of 800 mg a day will reduce the number of attacks considerably. Do not let genital herpes reduce your self-esteem: you are a worth-while person.

8. About syphilis

Syphilis is an infectious disease which is spread by sexual contact, so that it is contagious as well as infectious.

How likely is a person to get syphilis if he or she has sex with an infected partner? The exact chance is not easy to determine, but it seems that you have one chance in two of catching syphilis if you have sex with a person who has infectious syphilis in its two early stages. And, of course, the more times you have sex with him, or her, the greater is your chance of getting syphilis.

Syphilis is caused by a tiny slender corkscrew-shaped organism, which is invisible to the naked eye. It measures about 20 micrometres (μm) in length. A micrometre is one-thousandth of a millimetre in length, so that 500 organisms placed end to end would be needed to measure one centimetre, or 1250 to measure an inch. The organism is called *Treponema pallidum*, and it is coiled along its 20μm length. Usually there are about twelve coils. The *Treponema pallidum* can only live in the moist warm atmosphere of the human body, and dies within a very few hours outside it. But once inside the body it thrives.

If a person has a syphilitic ulcer on his or her genitals and has sexual contact with another person, the chance of acquiring syphilis is great. The surface of the ulcer contains millions of treponemes, and during sexual contact, 1000 or more are transferred to the other person's body through tiny invisible breaks in the skin or mucous membrane that comes into contact with the ulcer. Within 36 hours of being infected the number of treponemes doubles, and doubles again every 30 hours. By the time the person realizes that something is wrong, at least 10 000 million treponemes are in the person's body.

Within 30 minutes of being infected, the treponemes spread to the lymph nodes in the groins, where they are held up for a short time.

They then invade the bloodstream, and are carried throughout the body. Without treatment the organisms chronically infect almost all the tissues of the body and over the years invade and damage them.

However, the organisms do not have it all their own way. The *Treponema pallidum* has a fatty shell, but inside it contains protein. When a 'foreign' protein is injected into, or inoculated into, the body (as is the case of infection by syphilis) the body reacts. The foreign protein stimulates certain blood cells to multiply, and these cells are sensitized to the particular protein, so that should a further infection occur they mobilize to attack the invader at its point of entry, rather in the way in which a country attacked by a foreign invader tries to immobilize the invading army on the beaches. Unfortunately in the first, or primary, infection by syphilis the body's defences are inadequate, and the treponemes are not contained, so that they get into the bloodstream and multiply rapidly.

It takes about 3 weeks for the defences to be mobilized, which is why a person who has been infected with syphilis has no symptoms or signs for 3 weeks. Then the sensitized blood cells attack the treponemes, which are still multiplying in the tissues of the beach-head – in this case the mucous membrane of the penis or the vulva. This causes the first sign of syphilis, the raised pimple which appears on the vulva or penis. In the next few days many of the treponemes are killed, as are many of the white blood cells, with the result that a zone of hard tissue develops around the pimple. It also leads to a reduction in blood supply to the pimple, so that its centre dies and sloughs off, leaving an ulcer. In time the ulcer heals, leaving a scar. This takes from 3 to 8 weeks. Unfortunately, in some cases the primary lesion, the ulcer, is quite small, or is not even noticed, so that the infected person does not seek treatment. Usually the development of the genital ulcer induces the person to seek medical help. The doctor looks at the ulcer, which has firm edges and a soft centre, so that it resembles a button felt through a layer of cloth. It is called a hard chancre. From the raw, ulcerated centre clear fluid oozes. The fluid is infected with the treponemes. The lymph nodes in the area, usually those in the groin, will probably have become swollen and they feel like small round pieces of rubber under the skin.

The doctor cleanses the ulcer with a weak salt solution, then squeezes each side of it until clear fluid wells up from its red base. A sample of the fluid is placed between two glass slides and examined under a microscope with dark-ground illumination.

Viewed through a microscope with dark-ground illumination, the treponemes (which are also called spirochaetes) are seen as cork-screw-shaped organisms, which glisten bluish-white as they move, twisting on themselves (Fig. 8/1). Occasionally they bend on themselves and then snap straight. Occasionally their coils contract and then expand so that they look like animated watch springs.

During the period that the chancre is developing, the treponemes that have invaded the bloodstream cause another reaction. They induce the blood to make a chemical substance called an antibody. The formation of antibody to the treponemes is a slow process but, 4 to 8 weeks after the primary infection, it can be measured by taking a sample of blood from a vein. Two blood tests are usually made to detect syphilis. The first 'screening' test is called the Venereal Disease Research Laboratory Test (VDRL) and the second, the Treponema Pallidum Haemagglutination Test (TPHA). Both are equally effective in detecting syphilis but neither is specific for syphilis. For this reason if the VDRL or the TPHA test is positive a

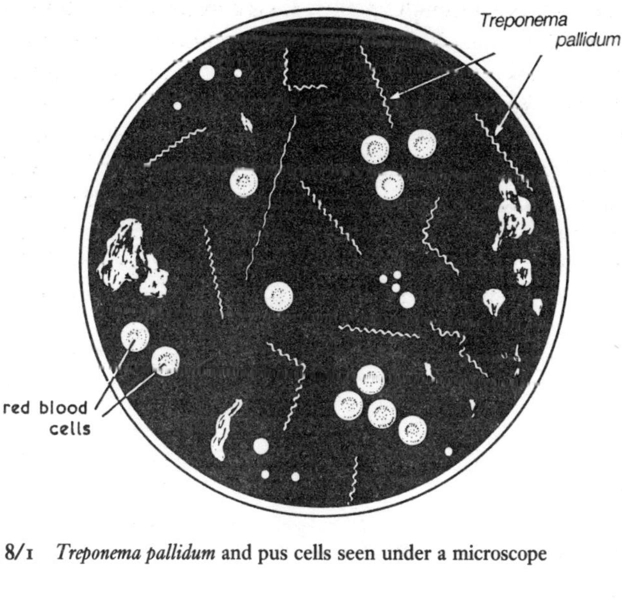

Fig. 8/1 *Treponema pallidum* and pus cells seen under a microscope

second more precise test (the FTA–ABS (fluorescent treponemal antibody absorption) test) is made to diagnose syphilis. Once formed, the antibody to syphilis tends to persist for years unless the syphilis is cured, when it usually disappears from the blood over a period of about a year. The measurement of the antibody by the VDRL test or its equivalent is the basis of the blood test to detect syphilis, which many states in the USA insist on making before a couple get married. This test is also made in early pregnancy to make sure that the expectant mother is not carrying syphilis in her blood, which may infect her unborn infant. It should also be made on all sexual contacts (who can be traced) to find how many of them have developed syphilis.

Syphilis is a sexually transmitted disease and since most couples have genital sex, which implies that the man's penis is inserted into the woman's vagina, the primary lesion of syphilis, the chancre, usually develops on the penis or on the woman's vulva (Figs 8/2 and 8/3). However, in about 25 per cent of women who are infected by a man with untreated syphilis, the primary lesion develops on the cervix and is invisible, but highly infectious should she have sexual

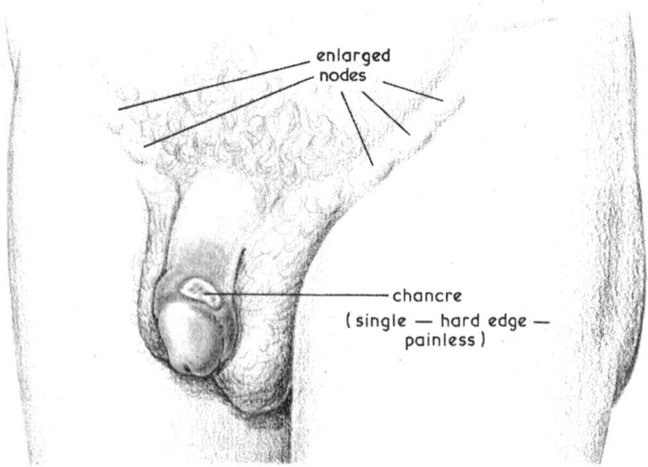

Fig. 8/2 The primary lesion of syphilis in a man – a chancre on the penis, with enlarged nodes in the groin

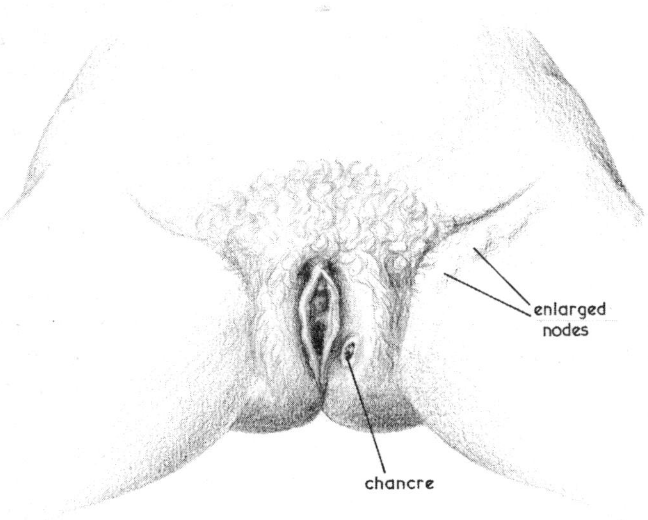

Fig. 8/3 The primary lesion of syphilis in a woman – a chancre on a labium, with enlarged nodes in the groin

intercourse with another, uninfected partner. Without treatment, the person who has syphilis remains infectious for about 2 years, after which the chance diminishes and it is unusual for an untreated syphilitic to transmit the disease after 5 years have passed. But, as will be seen, the disease continues to infect and to damage tissues in the body.

In 5 per cent of cases of primary syphilis, the lesion develops elsewhere than on the genitalia. Homosexuals who enjoy anal sex, if infected by a homosexual partner, may develop the chancre on the anus or in the lower part of the rectum. Couples, whether homo- or heterosexual, who enjoy oral sex may develop the lesion on the lips, or tongue, if either partner is infectious.

Very rarely, syphilis is acquired by means other than sexual intercourse. But these infections are so rare that in general they can be disregarded. Since the treponeme is so fragile when outside the human body and dies so rapidly, the story that you can pick up syphilis from a toilet seat is untrue. An elderly professor of medicine whom I once knew was asked by a student if you can get syphilis in a lavatory. 'Yes,' he replied, 'you can, but it is a ridiculous and improper place in which to have sexual intercourse.'

Syphilis is a chronic disease which, in the course of its untreated history, can infect almost any tissue of the body. For the understanding of the disease it is customary to divide it into three stages: primary, secondary and tertiary (or late), syphilis.

Primary stage

Primary syphilis is the stage of the initial infection and is first diagnosed clinically when the primary lesion, or chancre, appears 10 to 90 days after the person is infected. Most chancres develop in the period 20 to 25 days after sexual intercourse with an infected partner. The primary lesion has been described already, but it is worth repeating that it usually develops on the penis or the vulva, is usually single, has a hard edge and ulcerated centre from which clear fluid oozes, and is painless. It is extremely infectious. A few days after the appearance of the primary lesion, the lymph nodes in each groin enlarge to form painless rubbery masses. The primary lesion, if untreated, heals slowly over 4 to 8 weeks usually leaving a small scar.

Throughout this time the treponemes in the blood have been multiplying and have been provoking the reaction of the body's defences. As the antibody defence is provoked, the level of antibody in the blood rises. When the primary lesion has been present for 3 weeks, about 50 per cent of people tested will have a positive blood test; by 5 weeks, 80 per cent will have a positive test and by 10 weeks, if treatment has not been given, nearly all infected persons will have a positive blood test.

Secondary stage

6 to 8 weeks after the primary lesion, the secondary stage of syphilis develops. Quite often the infected person feels 'off colour', and may have headaches, fever, sore throat or joint pains, although these symptoms are not very helpful in making a diagnosis. There are four main groups of lesions that suggest secondary syphilis, and all of the secondary lesions are very infectious. By the time they appear, the blood tests for syphilis have become positive in over 99 per cent of

patients, so that diagnosis is easy if the patient is honest and helpful and the doctor alert.

The most common condition is a skin rash. More than 80 per cent of untreated patients have this. The rash starts as faint pale pink spots which appear first along the ribs and over the trunk but rapidly spreads, to cover the back and the belly, and appear on the face around the mouth and chin (Figs 8/4 and 8/5). Occasionally the rash forms a band across the forehead, which the doctors of the eighteenth century called 'the crown of Venus', in a whimsical, if accurate, way. The spots, which are usually round, rapidly become dusky red and as time passes may become pimply, and the centre of the pimple may shed its skin. They do not itch, but occasionally, if picked, become infected and form pus spots. The rash persists for about 6 weeks and then slowly fades, although it may reappear unless treatment has been given. In women, who sometimes have no visible primary lesions, the secondary skin rash may be the first sign to alert the doctor that the woman has syphilis.

The second common secondary lesion occurs in moist areas of the skin or on mucous membranes such as the mouth, the vulva and the anus. Because these areas are more delicate and moist, the second-

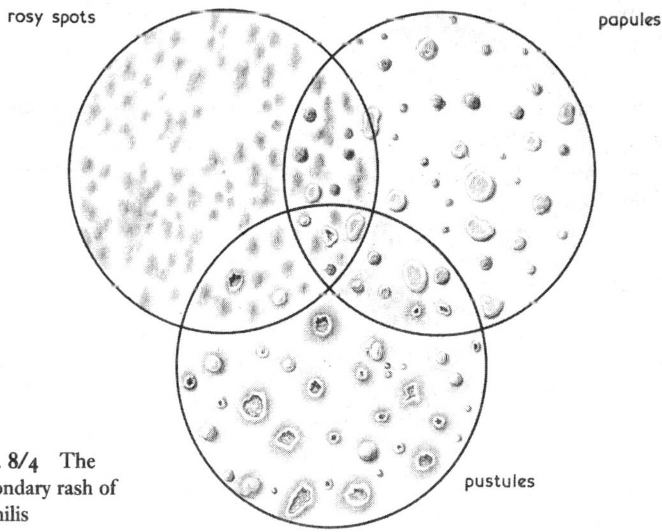

Fig. 8/4 The secondary rash of syphilis

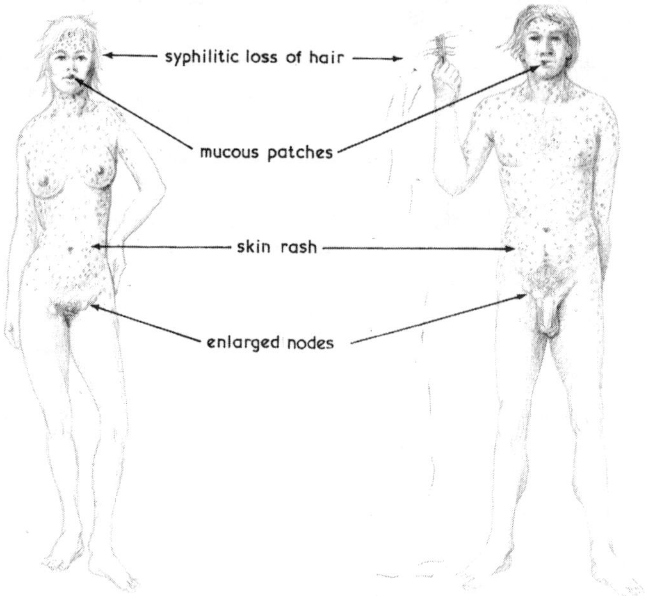

Fig. 8/5 The secondary stage of syphilis

ary lesions of syphilis that develop on them are different. In the vulval area in women, or around the anus in either sex (Fig. 8/6), warty growths may appear. These have flat tops and are reddish or grey in colour. They are very infectious, and occasionally appear in other moist areas, such as between the buttocks or on the scrotum. In the mouth, in the vagina, or on the penis, small grey raised patches, looking like snail tracks may develop. These, too, are painless and very infectious. They are called mucous patches (Fig. 8/7). Mucous patches and syphilitic warts affect about 30 per cent of untreated syphilitics.

The third finding is that many of the lymph nodes become swollen. These may be felt in the groins, armpits or the neck. Finally a few infected people develop signs of meningitis with irritating, recurrent headaches.

The secondary lesions of syphilis last from 3 to 12 months and then disappear.

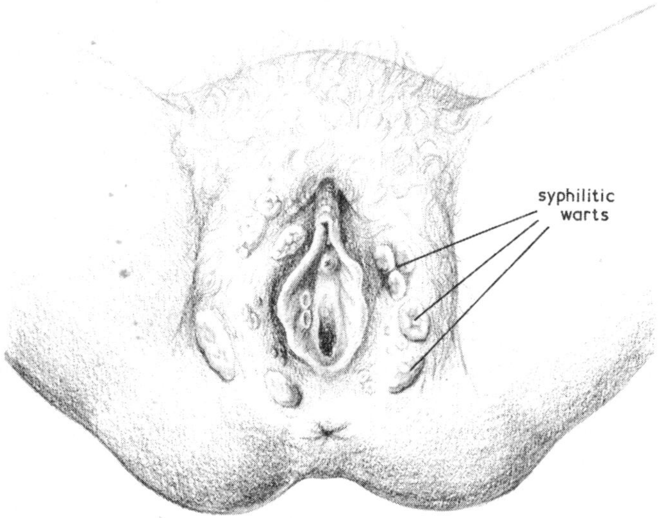

Fig. 8/6 Syphilitic warts on the vulva

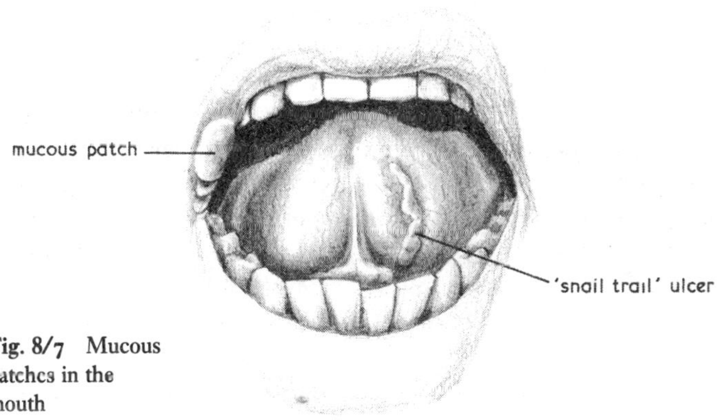

Fig. 8/7 Mucous patches in the mouth

Tertiary (third) stage

The third stage of syphilis may develop from 2 to 20 years after the disappearance of the secondary lesions. During this time the only indication that the patient has syphilis is that the blood test is positive. In many untreated patients the third stage fails to develop, although the person is at greater risk of dying than an uninfected person. Today, with effective treatment of early infectious syphilis, the lesions of the tertiary stage are increasingly less commonly encountered. In fact, we would not really know what happens to the untreated syphilitic were it not for a study in Oslo.

In 1891, Professor Brøck of Oslo, Norway, became convinced that the then current treatment of syphilis did nothing to cure the disease. At that time reliance was placed on mercury, which had first been suggested as a cure five centuries earlier. Mercury had been used for the treatment of leprosy since the twelfth century when it had been brought back from Palestine by the Crusaders. Used as an ointment – it was called Saracen's ointment – it was rubbed into the skin. It was not very effective in curing leprosy. As the manifestations of late syphilis resembled those of leprosy, so that the two diseases were often confused, mercury was introduced in the late 1400s for the treatment of syphilis. Four centuries later it was still the mainstay of treatment and, as Professor Brøck observed, it was almost useless. In fact he argued that the toxic side-effects of mercury were so many, and the cure of syphilis by using mercury so uncertain, that the effects of the treatment were worse than those of the disease.

He decided, therefore, not to treat any patients who developed syphilis, but because he knew the disease was highly infectious in the early stages, he kept them in hospital until all traces of syphilis had disappeared. This took from 3 to 12 months. After that time the patients were free to go about their business, but were expected to keep in contact with him for the rest of their lives. In all, he gave no treatment to nearly 2000 patients over the 20-year period up to 1910. By then, Paul Ehrlich had invented his 'magic bullet' against syphilis, which he called '606', or salvarsan. As it contained arsenic, not mercury, Professor Brøck felt that he had to discontinue his experiment, and to use salvarsan on all new patients. But he continued to follow up his old, untreated patients.

The follow-up through life, and by autopsy after death, of Professor Brøck's patients shows the natural history of syphilis. The first observation was that in 24 per cent of the patients, a relapse occurred after the secondary lesions had cleared. The relapse occurred within 2 years of the primary infection in most patients, and 55 of the 244 patients who had one relapse had a second relapse.

The nature of the relapse was that the lesions in the moist areas recurred, mainly in the mouth, in the throat, or around the anus. During the relapse the patient again became highly infectious to others. And then, for no reason, in about 3 to 6 months, the ulcers disappeared and the patient was again cured.

The remainder of the observations were about late, or tertiary, syphilis. These were made by Professor Brøck's successor, Dr Bruusgaard, and by his successor, Dr Danbolt. A total of 953 patients were followed to their death, or at least for 40 years after they were first infected (Fig. 8/8). Of these, 60 per cent had no further clinical evidence of the disease, although the treponemes were insidiously damaging their tissues. This is shown by mortality, or death, statistics.

The syphilitic patients had a greater chance of dying at an earlier

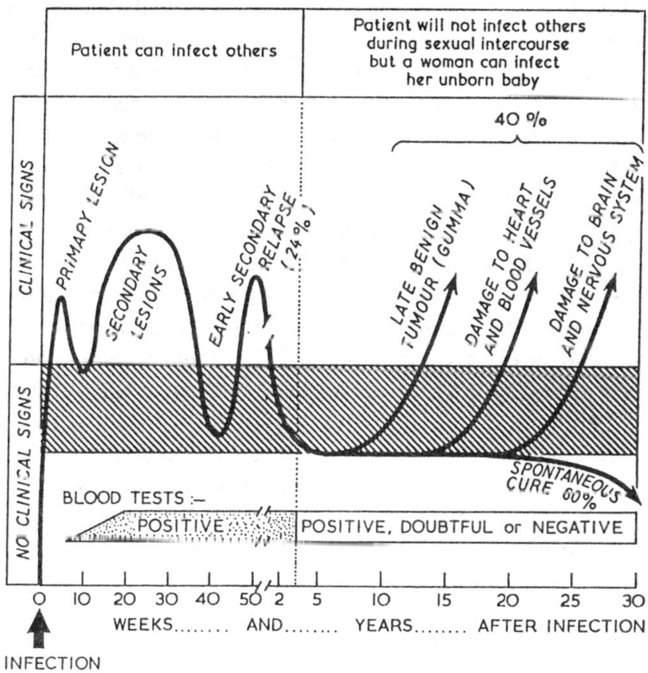

Fig. 8/8 The natural history of untreated syphilis

age than non-syphilitic people. Death was more likely to occur to men between the ages of 40 and 49, when the extra chance of dying was 122 per cent higher than that of non-syphilitics; and to women between the ages of 30 and 49, when their extra chance of dying, over non-syphilitic women of a similar age, was 90 per cent. But at all ages the chance of death occurring to a syphilitic person was greater than to a non-syphilitic person. The untreated disease shortened a person's life, even if syphilis was not the cause of death. In fact syphilis was the direct cause of death in only one patient in ten.

Signs of late syphilis developed in 40 per cent of the untreated patients. These showed in three ways. In 15 per cent of cases, the patient developed a thickened ulcerating tumour in or under the skin or in a bone. If the tumour, which was called a gumma, developed in the skin, the skin rotted away leaving a painful ulcer, which usually became infected (Fig. 8/9). If the gumma developed in a bone, usually a bone of the lower leg, or the skull, the patient complained of a deep, gnawing boring pain which was worse at night and went on and on.

In about 10 per cent of the cases, damage to the heart or great blood vessels appeared from 10 to 30 years after the primary infection. This form of the disease affected men twice as often as women, and was thought to occur more frequently among heavy manual workers. If the heart was affected, the patient developed

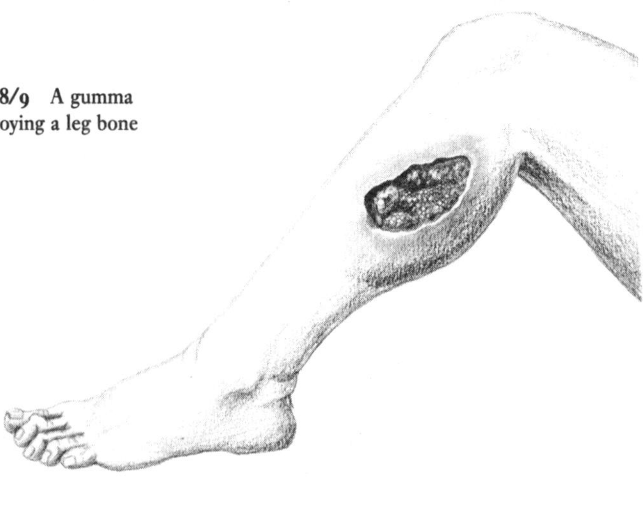

Fig. 8/9 A gumma destroying a leg bone

chest pain and shortness of breath. If the great vessels were affected he or she often had no symptoms, but was likely to drop dead suddenly when the aorta ruptured.

A further 10 per cent of the Oslo patients developed syphilis of the brain or spinal cord. This occurred from 5 to 35 years after the initial infection. Once again, more men than women were affected in this particularly horrible way. The disease showed as mental decay and, at autopsy, the brain of the victim was shrunken. First the person's memory worsened, then his concentration became less and he developed a lack of judgement. Then, in succession, he lost emotional control, so that he would fall into episodes of weeping, or of rage, for no reason. Finally he developed delusions, either of grandeur or of guilt, or he became demented and apathetic.

If the spinal cord was affected, he developed tabes dorsalis, when he had fleeting sharp pains in his shins, as if someone had beaten his legs with the back of an axe; and he developed an unsteady swaying gait which was worse at night. Both of these symptoms progressed as the years went by, until the patient was able to walk only with the help of a stick and eventually became bedridden, incontinent of urine and sometimes blind. In the last stages, violent episodes of gut pain and vomiting occurred, as did severe pain in the rectum, in the bladder, or in the penis.

A similar study took place between 1930 and 1950 in Tuskegee County in Alabama. The findings were similar to those of the Norwegian study.

Today, with adequate treatment of the early stages of syphilis, the third-stage lesions are increasingly rare, but they cause so much misery that a person who thinks he might have syphilis should be tested. If he is found to have the disease, he should be treated adequately, so that he infects no other person, and so that he avoids the lesions of tertiary syphilis, and the greater likelihood of premature death which affects the untreated syphilitic.

Prenatal syphilis

Syphilis can be transmitted from an infected woman to her unborn baby long after she has ceased to be able to transmit the disease to men during sexual intercourse. This is because the treponemes continue to multiply in her bloodstream. But it is also true that the more recently she has acquired syphilis, the greater is the chance that her unborn baby will be affected. The treponemes manage to penetrate the placenta, or afterbirth, which separates the baby from its mother, and then infect the baby. Because of the character of the placenta, penetration occurs only in the second half of pregnancy, after the end of the 20th week from the time of the last menstrual period. This means that if blood tests are made in the first 10 weeks of pregnancy on all pregnant women, those women who have had syphilis which was not properly treated, and those who have contracted syphilis and do not know it, can be treated with penicillin before the baby is affected. This means that the baby will be completely healthy.

In most developed (Western) countries all pregnant women are routinely tested for syphilis. Fortunately the number of women who have syphilis is few and in Britain, for example, only 1 in every 2000 antenatal patients has a positive test. But the test is worth doing because of the damage untreated syphilis causes to the unborn baby and because the baby is the innocent victim of its mother's disease. About a quarter of infected unborn babies die in the womb and the mother delivers a dead, swollen, skin-peeling, bloated baby. The remaining 75 per cent of infected babies are born alive, but a quarter die early in life if no treatment is given. Of the remainder, half develop the signs of tertiary syphilis between the ages of 7 and 15.

The progress of the disease in the infant is the same as that in the infected adult. The primary stage takes place while the baby is in its mother's womb. The secondary stage is present at birth or becomes noticeable within 6 weeks of birth. The skin rashes are particularly common and highly infectious (Fig. 8/10), but the infant's nose and throat may be affected and mucous patches may develop, so that the child whines and snuffles. A few infants develop swellings in the ends of their bones, especially the long bones of their legs. If the leg is moved the child screams with pain. In 10 per cent of children infected in the womb, the treponemes invade the child's brain, and this may lead to convulsions and mental deficiency.

If the infant is treated in early life it will be cured; but if it is not, tertiary syphilis may develop when the child is aged between 7 and 15. Rarely it occurs earlier, or later in adult life. As in the adult, three

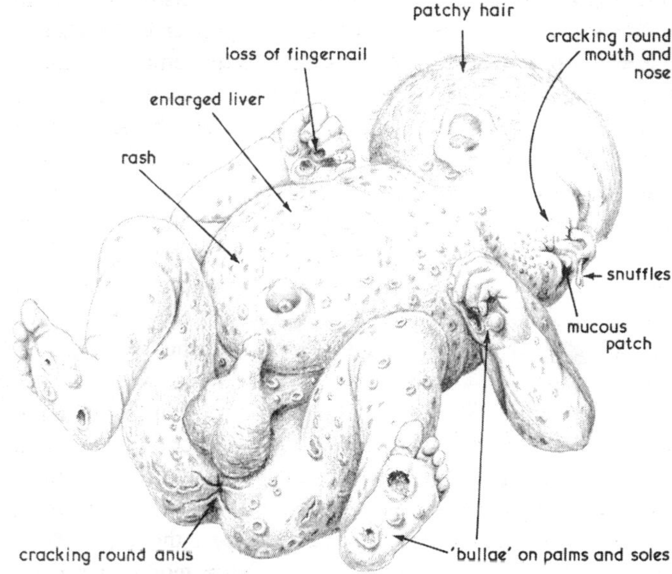

Fig. 8/10 Prenatal syphilitic infection

lesions are common. The first are gummas which form especially in the cartilage of the child's nose, or the palate of his mouth, and may cause collapse of the bridge of the nose. They also tend to develop in the bones of the lower leg. This causes a painful swelling and deformity of the leg. In 25 to 50 per cent of prenatally infected children, the disease damages the cornea of the eyes. It starts with pain in the eye, particularly when the child looks at a bright light, and he or she complains of mistiness of vision. The episode lasts for a few weeks and then goes. The attacks recur, and with each attack the child's sight is diminished, so that blindness eventually occurs.

Finally, between 10 and 15 per cent of untreated prenatally infected syphilitics develop mental damage, with the mental changes already described.

The tragedy of the so-called 'congenital' syphilitic (that is, the child infected while still in the womb) is that the disease is entirely preventable. If every pregnant woman had a blood test taken for syphilis at least once in pregnancy, and if every woman with a positive test was treated with penicillin injections, 'congenital' syphilis would disappear. In fact, in the developed nations, 'congenital' syphilis is increasingly rare, but it does occur. It should not.

Treatment of syphilis

Today, the chances of curing early syphilis, that is syphilis in the first or second stage, are excellent. And even in the third stage, the disease can be arrested, although not cured.

The discovery of penicillin and of the other antibiotics has completely changed the outlook. But it is not enough for an infected person to receive a full course of penicillin. He or she must also be prepared to have blood tests made at periodic intervals to make sure that a relapse does not occur. Because of the gross damage that syphilis may cause to a person's body and mind, the follow-up has to be even more scrupulous than that following treatment for gonorrhoea.

Usually, daily injections of penicillin are given, together with probenecid tablets to maintain high blood levels of the antibiotic for 10 days. If it is thought that the infected person is likely to fail to turn up each day, a single injection of a form of penicillin (benzathine penicillin) is given as a single dose into a muscle. For people who are allergic to penicillin, oxytetracycline 500mg (2 capsules) are taken 4 times a day for 15 days.

Following the treatment, the patient is examined and blood tests are taken every month for 6 months, and then again at 9 months and 12 months, after the initial treatment. If the tests are negative by the end of the year, the patient is considered cured.

If syphilis is not detected until the end of or after the secondary stage, the treatment is the same, but the follow-up tests are made every 2 months for the first year, and then every 3 months for a second year.

In both early infective, and later latent syphilis, the blood tests may show the need for further injections of penicillin.

The person who has acquired syphilis must obviously co-operate with the health professionals in his or her treatment and must attend when requested for tests. Failure to do this in the early stages may lead to infection of others, and in the latter stages poses a danger to the person herself or himself.

9. About human immunodeficiency virus (HIV) infection – AIDS

AIDS is caused by a virus which is usually sexually transmitted, but may be spread if drug addicts share infected needles. In the past, a few cases of AIDS occurred some time after a person had received an infected blood transfusion. This occurrence is now extremely rare.

The AIDS virus was identified in France and in the USA at about the same time. Each country had its own name for the virus, but in 1985 an international group of scientists decided that the virus should be called the human immunodeficiency virus or HIV.

HIV seems to be a relatively new virus and the first cases of AIDS were diagnosed in Central Africa. In Africa, HIV infection and AIDS is predominantly a sexually transmitted disease acquired from prostitutes. Between 5 and 25 per cent of sexually active adults in the urban populations of several African countries have been infected with the HIV virus. Between 70 and 80 per cent of them will probably develop AIDS.

In 1981, AIDS was diagnosed in the USA, and the next year in European countries and in Australasia. The diagnosis of AIDS was first made when a number of homosexual men developed a severe pneumonia, prolonged unexplained fever, or a rare cancer called Kaposi's sarcoma. These severe illnesses were often accompanied by severe fungal or parasitic infections. The bizarre nature of the illnesses and their multiple forms led to intensive investigations. These disclosed that an infected person's resistance to all infections was considerably diminished because his immune system was damaged. The damage particularly affected the helper T-cells, which were reduced in number with the consequence that the person could not resist infection by bacteria, fungi or other viruses as successfully as a non-infected person (Fig. 9/1). In other words the

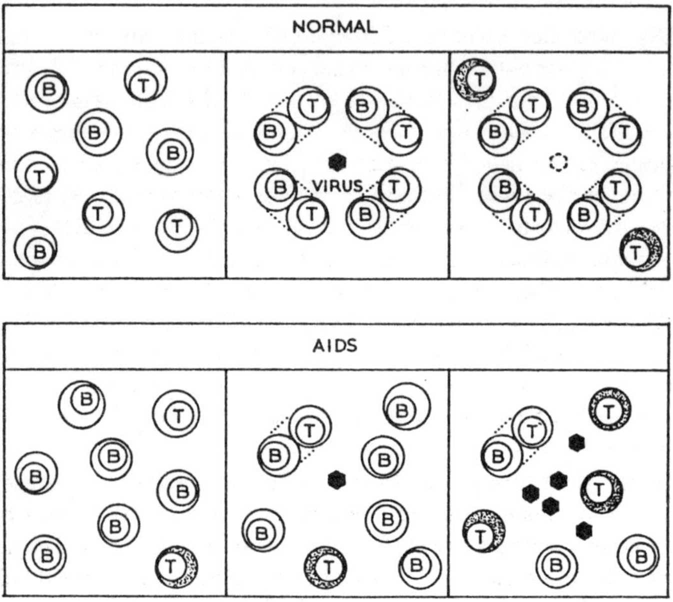

Fig. 9/1 The immune system in health and in AIDS.

Normal

1. White blood cells called lymphocytes act like an army, rallying the body's defences against invading micro-organisms which cause infection. One type of lymphocyte, the B cell, produces antibodies to attack the invading germs; and another type of lymphocyte, the T cells, are produced by a gland in the neck, called the thymus gland (hence T cell). Two kinds of T cells are produced, 'helper' cells and 'suppressor' cells.
2. In a healthy person the helper cells assist the B cells in their attack on the virus.
3. The suppressor cells (shown as shaded) help call off the attack. In healthy people there are about two helper cells for every one suppressor cell.

AIDS

4. People who have acquired AIDS lose their ability to fight severe infections because the virus damages their helper T cells.
5. This means that AIDS victims produce far fewer helper cells and so have fewer T cells to protect them against infection.
6. In AIDS victims, the ratio between helper and suppressor cells is reversed; with three suppressors to every one helper. Their bodies have given up the fight against infection before it begins

person had become immunodeficient, hence the name the Acquired Immune Deficiency Syndrome or AIDS.

As mentioned earlier HIV infection is usually transmitted from one person to another during sexual contact in which the HIV virus in the infected person's blood, semen or vaginal secretions enters the partner's body. During sexual intercourse, tiny tears and abrasions, invisible to the naked eye, may occur in the surface lining of the rectum or the vagina because of the thrusting movements of the penis. Damage to the rectum is more likely to occur than damage to the vagina, because the lining is more delicate, so that rectal intercourse is more likely to lead to infection by HIV.

Although the virus has been detected in several body fluids, it is not transmitted by contact with tears, or spread by sneezing, coughing or spitting. It is not spread by social kissing, although it may be spread by deep kissing and by oral sex if one partner is infected.

In the USA, Europe, and Australasia, over 75 per cent of those infected are homosexual or bisexual men, particularly those who have several partners and prefer anal intercourse. The second group of people who are at greater risk of being infected are drug addicts who mainline and share needles. HIV infection and AIDS is not contracted by swimming in a pool in which a person infected with HIV has swum, or from eating in a restaurant used by an AIDS patient. AIDS is not contracted by sharing eating utensils, towels or bed linen with an infected person. You cannot get infected by HIV if you use a toilet, or a telephone used by an infected person. A person cannot be infected during body massage or other body contacts that do not include sexual intercourse or oral sex. Oral sex is an unusual way of getting HIV infection; most people are infected after anal, or less commonly, vaginal sex.

It must be stressed that HIV infection and AIDS is not a homosexual disease. AIDS affects heterosexual men and women. AIDS affects children.

A group of women who need some consideration are pregnant women who are infected with the AIDS virus. Although HIV infection does not affect the progress of the pregnancy adversely, between 20 and 40 per cent of the babies will be infected inside the uterus. When they are born they will be HIV positive and will develop AIDS. Pregnant women who are HIV positive should consider seriously requesting an abortion. Women who are at risk of being infected with HIV should be tested for infection either before they decide to become pregnant or in early pregnancy.

There is a very slight chance that a mother who has been infected with HIV may infect her baby through her breast milk. This must be taken into consideration if the infected woman chooses to continue with the pregnancy, or if pregnancy is diagnosed too late for an abortion.

In the recent past a number of people became infected with the virus from an infected blood transfusion. Today the risk of this occurring is minimal, probably less than one chance in 100 000 blood transfusions. This is because both the donors and the donated blood are tested carefully to make sure that no contamination with HIV has occurred.

The test is made by examining the blood to make sure that it does not contain any antibodies to the HIV. The antibodies to the HIV are detected by a test called Elisa. As other infections may lead to a positive Elisa test, the Elisa test is a 'screening test' and a further test is made if the Elisa test is positive. This is a specific test for the HIV called Western Blot. It takes 2 weeks to obtain the result.

The tests are also made to find out if a person has been infected with the HIV. However, they do not become positive immediately after the person is infected. There is a delay of 3 weeks to 3 months. In the interval between being infected with HIV and the appearance in the person's blood of the antibodies, the person is very infectious. If a person has a positive Elisa test for HIV which is confirmed by the Western Blot test, he or she is infected with HIV and should avoid having sexual intercourse with an uninfected person, unless the man wears a condom. He or she should also avoid contaminating another person with his or her blood, particularly by sharing needles for injecting drugs.

Most people infected with the AIDS virus have no symptoms and feel well for months or years. But after an interval of between 3 and 14 years between 30 and 50 per cent of them will develop the second stage of AIDS, the AIDS Related Complex, and between 7 and 15 per cent will develop 'full-blown AIDS'. By 15 years after being infected it is believed that over three quarters of those infected will have 'full-blown AIDS'.

It is not known why some people remain well and why the disease progresses in others. Research has shown that progress is more likely if the person acquires another sexually transmitted disease, such as NGGI or gonorrhoea. Another factor seems to be if the person continues to practise anal intercourse. If the disease progresses, the person will feel 'off-colour', be easily fatigued, start losing weight, have unexplained sweating attacks and swollen glands which persist for some time. These symptoms make up the clinical appearance of the second stage of AIDS, the AIDS Related Complex (ARC).

Between 15 and 30 per cent of those who have ARC will develop 'full-blown' AIDS in 9 to 30 months, and more will develop it as time passes.

The third stage of AIDS – 'full-blown AIDS' – is a terrifying disease. The person feels increasingly unwell, always tired and often depressed. Many victims develop a severe form of pneumonia or other 'opportunistic' infections, and more than 60 per cent die, on average 13 months after the infection is first diagnosed. Other infected people develop Kaposi's sarcoma. If this occurs the person has a 50 per cent chance of dying within 21 months after diagnosis. If the person develops both an opportunistic infection and Kaposi's sarcoma death is quicker. In addition the virus affects the brain, the infected person becoming mentally disturbed, depressed, or apathetic.

There is no cure for AIDS and as yet no vaccine to prevent the infection occurring. However, there is hope for some sufferers in the symptomless stage of AIDS. If the person takes small doses of the drug zidovudine (AZT), progress of the disease may be delayed as long as he or she continues taking the drug. The number of helper T-cells increases, and the person is better able to resist infections. Zidovudine also reduces the severity of the disease and prolongs the life of sufferers who have 'full-blown' AIDS. In the doses required to help people with full-blown AIDS there are some side-effects, such as nausea, muscle pains and headaches, but the severity of these can be reduced by other treatment.

In 1988 the World Health Organization adopted a more complete classification of infection with HIV. It is as follows:

Group 1. Initial acute infection. The person feels unwell, may have a fever, and thinks he has a 'virus'. This lasts about a week.

Group 2. Asymptomatic infection. The person feels well, but the virus is growing in his blood and he may infect another with whom he has anal or vaginal intercourse.

Group 3. Persistent generalized lymphadenopathy. The person develops a long-lasting swelling of his lymph glands, but has no other symptoms.

Group 4. Full-blown AIDS. This is divided into several groups depending on the predominant symptoms.

The first group are people who have fevers, night sweats, weight loss and diarrhoea. These were previously diagnosed as having ARC.

The second group are those people who have brain symptoms. The symptoms are those of early dementia. The person's attention span, memory, understanding and motor coordination are impaired.

The third group are those people who develop opportunistic infections such as pneumonia and severe candidal infection.

The fourth group are those people who develop cancers such as Kaposi's sarcoma.

A fifth group are those who develop the AIDS wasting disease.

As mentioned, the health of most people who have full-blown AIDS deteriorates over time and eventually most will die. As the person becomes increasingly ill, he or she becomes weaker, and often depressed and confused. During these months he or she needs support, love and help from family, from a lover or from a friend. As death nears some may choose to go into hospital, others may wish to remain at home, amongst familiar surroundings, until they are so ill that admission to hospital is imperative. In most countries, comfort, support and love can be given to the dying by dedicated trained volunteers. In the USA the 'buddy system' was started. In Australia, the support system is called Ankali, from an aboriginal word meaning 'friend'. The carer is just that: a person who provides companionship, love and help to the victim and, above all, is there when needed. The carer listens to and talks with the dying person, when that person wants someone to talk to. The carer does not counsel, nor does he or she offer treatment.

At the present time (1990) it has been estimated that over 350 000 people in the world have ARC or full-blown AIDS. The numbers are rising as those who have symptomless HIV infection develop symptoms. It is believed that there are 25 people infected with HIV to each case of ARC or full-blown AIDS, so that there are at least 8.5 million HIV-infected people in the world.

As AIDS cannot be cured at present, the epidemic which is currently sweeping the world will only be controlled if people change their sexual (and drug abuse) behaviours. Safer sex will limit the spread of the HIV virus and hence of AIDS. Safer sex means avoiding sex with several partners, particularly if you are homosexual and practise anal sex. Safer sex means that unless you know with reasonable certainty that your partner has not been infected with the HIV, you should make sure that condoms are used during anal or vaginal intercourse. To some extent this is already occurring. Information from Sweden and Britain shows that since 1983 the number of men and women infected with gonorrhoea or syphilis is falling, suggesting that safer sex is being practised, and an increasing number of homosexual men are practising safer sex.

The second way of reducing the spread of the HIV virus is to make sure that intravenous drug addicts do not share needles. One of the ways of achieving this objective is to provide sterile needles to registered drug addicts or to make them readily and cheaply available at pharmacist's shops.

One special group of people require further consideration. These are the health workers who care for AIDS victims. Although health workers have a slightly greater risk of being infected with the HIV, the risk is very small if they take the following precautions:

* Take extreme care to avoid accidental wounds from sharp instruments contaminated with potentially infectious material and to avoid exposing open skin lesions to material from AIDS patients.
* If the health worker is accidentally injured by a needle (needle-stick injury) persuade the patient to be tested for HIV infection, if his or her HIV status is not known.

* Wear gloves when handling blood specimens, blood-soiled items, body fluids, excretions and secretions, as well as when handling surfaces, materials, and objects exposed to such fluids.
* Wear gowns when clothing may be soiled with body fluids, blood, secretions or excretions.
* Wash hands after removing gowns and gloves before leaving the rooms of known or suspected AIDS patients; wash immediately if contaminated with blood.
* Label blood and other specimens prominently with a special warning, such as 'AIDS PRECAUTIONS'.
* Place blood-soiled articles from an AIDS patient in an impervious bag, prominently labelled 'AIDS PRECAUTIONS', before sending them for reprocessing or disposal.
* Do not bend needles after use, but place promptly in a puncture-resistant container for disposal. Do not re-insert used needles into their original sheaths before discarding, as this is a common cause of needle injury.
* Use disposable syringes and needles.
* Request a private room for patients too ill to use good hygiene.

Surgeons and their assistants during operations are at greater risk of being infected, because surgical operations are usually accompanied by some spurting of blood and because of the danger of needle-stick injury. Many surgeons now expect all patients who need surgery to be tested for HIV infection so that the surgical team can take additional precautions to avoid being infected. This is being opposed by some civil libertarians as an invasion of the rights of the individual and because even with the most strict tests a few people are erroneously told that they have been infected with HIV. An agreed consensus is needed, to safeguard the rights of the surgical teams and those of the patients.

The psychological effects of HIV infection

The knowledge that a person has been infected with the HIV virus and that he or she is HIV positive causes an immense psychological upset. This is aggravated by the knowledge that most people infected with HIV will go on to develop the later stages of AIDS and that there is no cure, so that death is likely in 10 to 15 years. Society's condemnatory attitude to people infected with HIV and the discrimination against those people who let it be known that they are infected adds to the emotional turmoil. The psychological damage is further increased by the knowledge that the person's partner, male or female, is likely to be infected. The emotional distress may be so severe that thoughts of suicide are common, and some people infected commit suicide.

People infected by HIV need supportive counselling and the opportunity to talk with empathetic, non-judgemental helpers when problems arise. There is research evidence that the knowledge of being infected with HIV is as emotionally devastating as the knowledge that the person has full-blown AIDS.

10. About hepatitis

Viral hepatitis

Although not strictly a sexually transmitted disease, the virus which causes hepatitis A (HAV) and that which causes the more serious hepatitis B (HBV) may be transmitted from an infected partner during sexual intercourse. A third virus causes another form of hepatitis (called hepatitis non-A, non-B) but at present it is not known whether this virus is sexually transmitted.

HEPATITIS A

The virus causing hepatitis A is shed in an infected person's faeces in great quantities. Should the virus contaminate food, either because the person preparing the food transfers the virus from the anus to the hands and to the food, or if the food is contaminated by flies, another person eating the food may be infected. Transmission may also occur if a person has sex with an infected partner, particularly if oro-genital, anal or oro-anal sexual stimulation takes place.

About 30 days after infection, the person feels 'off-colour' and then a few days later jaundice occurs in adults, but many children who are infected show no symptoms. In countries with poor hygiene, almost all children have been infected, but in the developed countries only about 20 per cent have been infected. Once a person has been infected, antibodies develop which protect the person against further infections.

Hepatitis A is increasing among adults in the developed nations, many of the infections being brought back by returning travellers. Although an inconvenience, hepatitis A is a relatively benign disease.

HEPATITIS B

This is a much more serious illness which is spread in the same way as hepatitis A and has the same set of symptoms. The difference between the two forms is that some people who have had hepatitis B fail to eliminate the virus and become 'carriers'.

Carriers continue to have virus in their blood and to secrete it into their body secretions, especially those of the intestinal tract. The earlier in life a person is infected, the greater chance he or she has of becoming a carrier. If a carrier has close bodily contact with another person and especially if that contact involves oro-genital or anal sex, the sexual partner may develop hepatitis B.

Carriers can be detected by examining the blood for a special substance called hepatitis B surface antigen (HB_sAg). In most Western communities, fewer than 1 person in 100 has HB_sAg in their blood. Among Asians the proportion who have HB_sAg is about 15 per cent, and about 8 per cent of drug addicts are infected.

Because the baby of a woman carrier may be infected in the womb, in many countries all pregnant women are tested for HB_sAg. If the test is positive the baby is treated with gamma-globulin and hepatitis B vaccine soon after birth.

Promiscuous homosexual men are also more likely to be carriers of hepatitis B and may infect a sexual partner. This is the reason for including hepatitis B as a sexually transmitted disease.

Surveys in the USA show that about 10 per cent of promiscuous homosexual men have HB_sAg in their blood and are carriers. In Australia the proportion is lower, being about 5 per cent. In addition, promiscuous homosexual men have twice the chance of having acquired hepatitis (either A or B) at some time than heterosexual men. The more sexual partners a man has had, the higher the chance that he will have acquired hepatitis, and the higher the chance he will become a carrier. If he has had hepatitis, he has a one in five chance of having permanent liver damage, including cirrhosis of the liver.

For this reason a homosexual man would be wise to be checked by blood tests, first to find out if he is immune to hepatitis A and B and second to find out if he has HB_sAg in his blood and is a carrier who could infect a sexual partner. If he is a carrier he should avoid oral and anal sex until his partner has been given injections of hepatitis B vaccine, which will protect him against developing hepatitis B.

11. About the minor sexually transmitted diseases

The minor sexually transmitted diseases fall into two groups. The first group defines those diseases that cause vaginal infections and, less commonly, infect the man's penis. These include vaginal candida infections (previously called thrush and monilia), trichomoniasis and non-specific vaginitis. The second group of diseases affects both sexual partners equally. They include genital warts, pubic lice and molluscum contagiosum.

Vaginal infections

During a woman's reproductive years, from puberty to menopause, the lining of the vagina is between 10 and 30 cells thick. The cells, which are exposed to the interior of the vagina, are constantly shed, to be replaced by the next layer of cells. This process continues because the deepest cells are constantly dividing to produce the next layer. As the cells approach the surface, changes occur in them and these changes are determined by the quantity of oestrogen, the female sex hormone, circulating in the blood at the time. The cells nearest the surface have small nuclei, and the substance of each cell contains a quantity of the carbohydrate, glycogen.

When the cells are shed into the interior of the vagina, the glycogen is converted into lactic acid by bacteria which normally live there. The lactic acid reduces, or eliminates the growth of potentially harmful bacteria and so keeps the vagina clean. In addition to the acid-forming bacteria, the vagina harbours large numbers of other bacteria, which in most circumstances cause no problems. However, in certain circumstances, a change in vaginal acidity or resistance occurs and vaginal infection may result, either from an overgrowth of certain of the normal vaginal bacterial inhabitants or because organisms are introduced into the vagina during sexual intercourse.

Normally the vagina is kept moist by fluid which seeps through the vaginal walls from the blood vessels that surround it. The fluid mixes with the shed vaginal cells and is added to by secretions from the cervix and from Bartholin's glands. The quantity of the normal vaginal fluid varies considerably, and 'stress', anxiety, depression or an inadequate sexual relationship, seem to increase the amount. When this happens the woman notices an increased discharge, which may have a mild odour and which, on drying, leaves a stain on her panties or pantihose.

The vaginal discharge may worry the woman so much that she visits a doctor, fearing that she has a sexually transmitted disease. In most cases the doctor has to examine a sample of the discharge, smeared on a slide, under a microscope to make sure that the woman does not have one of the minor sexually transmitted diseases. As well as this, he may place a drop or two of the discharge on a slide and mix it with a drop or two of potassium hydroxide. He then smells the mixture. A strong fishy smell may indicate that the woman has non-specific vaginitis.

If these simple office tests fail to disclose the cause of the woman's vaginal discharge, the doctor takes a further vaginal swab and sends this to a laboratory for culture.

CANDIDIASIS (VAGINAL THRUSH OR MONILIA)

Depending on social class, age and sexual behaviour, between 5 and 30 per cent of women harbour the fungus, *Candida albicans*, in their vagina. The fungus usually causes no symptoms and the growth is kept in check by other vaginal bacteria. But if an event occurs that alters this balance, candida will start growing and may cause a vaginal inflammation.

For example, candidiasis is often found in diabetic women, and is particularly common in pregnancy. It may also cause symptoms after a woman has been given a course of penicillin, or some other antibiotic. A great deal of discussion has taken place to decide whether candidiasis is more likely to occur among women on the pill; and although it does appear to be more common, the evidence is by no means certain. It is better to be protected against an unwanted pregnancy by taking the pill than to worry about the chance of developing vaginal candidiasis.

Without contraception, pregnancy is more likely to follow and pregnancy is a particularly strong stimulus to the appearance of vaginal candidiasis. The pill is the most efficient of all the available contraceptives, and in most cases will be the first choice. But if a woman has had candidiasis previously, she may choose to have an intra-uterine device inserted into her uterus or to use a vaginal diaphragm. These methods do not give such good protection against unwanted pregnancy, but are still very efficient. Alternatively the woman's partner can use a condom, while she uses a spermicidal vaginal cream each time they have sexual intercourse.

Candida may also be introduced into a woman's vagina from the penis of a partner who has candidiasis; and the reverse may happen, the man complaining of an itchy penis after intercourse with an infected woman.

The statistics from several countries suggest that about a quarter of women who harbour candida develop symptoms at some time.

Candida albicans, so called to distinguish it from other forms of the fungus, is a yeast-like organism, which grows particularly well in a moist atmosphere, especially when the secretions contain carbohydrate. This fungus is the cause of candidiasis in over 90 per cent of women. If bacteria are present its growth tends to be suppressed, which is why it is more likely to grow when a woman has taken antibiotics to eliminate bacterial infection somewhere in her body.

The main symptom in women is an intense itching of the vagina and the vulva and this is associated with a thickish, whitish, non-smelly vaginal discharge, which is often profuse. The itch can be quite intolerable and is noticed particularly at night. If the woman scratches herself to relieve the itch, her vulva may become very sore and swollen. Occasionally scratching introduces secondary infection, and small, exquisitely painful ulcers result, with increased swelling of the labia around her vulva.

In men who are infected by sexual partners who harbour the fungus, the glans penis and the foreskin become itchy. Occasionally the condition leads to a urethral discharge. A few men develop small superficial ulcers on the glans penis 2 days or so after sexual

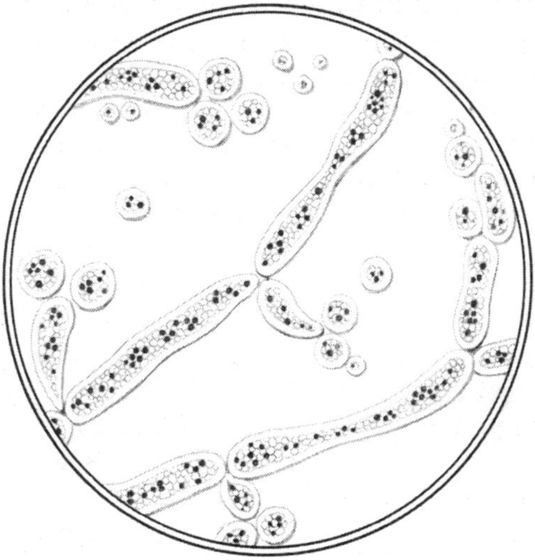

Fig. 11/1 *Candida albicans* seen through a microscope

intercourse. These are very itchy and are associated with a burning feeling over the glans penis.

The diagnosis may be easy, or rather difficult. In a typical case, a specimen of the discharge, placed on a glass slide and stained appropriately, shows the fungus as long threads with bulbous protuberances when viewed down a microscope (Fig. 11/1). In other cases the discharge has to be inoculated into a culture medium, and incubated for 48 hours before the fungus can be found. When the woman complains of very little vaginal discharge, but a very itchy vulva, tiny scrapings of skin taken painlessly from the vulva, and stained, may show *Candida albicans*.

In most cases of vaginal candidiasis treatment is relatively simple. The woman places a tablet (often called an 'ovule' because of its shape) or an applicator full of cream, high in her vagina for one or more nights, or twice a day for a number of days. The medication kills the fungus and is called a fungicide. The duration of the treatment varies depending on the fungicide chosen, and no one drug is better than any other. However, experience has shown that most women prefer fungicides which only need to be used for a short time. In addition the male partner may need to apply the fungicidal cream to his penis. The available fungicides, their trade names and the duration of treatment are shown in Table 11/1.

A few women are not so easily treated. In them the fungus causes such a marked reaction that it is difficult to use the pessaries, and the vulva may be so swollen and painful that sitting and sleeping are impossible. When this occurs, the woman needs to be admitted to hospital, so that soothing soaks can be applied to the inflamed vulva and the vagina can be painted with swabs dipped into the blue-coloured 'gentian violet'. This treatment is messy but effective, when the more specific treatment using one of the fungicides is not possible, or fails to cure the condition.

Persistent or frequently recurring vaginal candidiasis occurs in about 5 per cent of women. Recurrent candida infections are probably due to a failure of the body's immune system to eliminate the fungus which has entered the cells lining the vagina. Instead it lies dormant for a while and then multiplies, producing symptoms. It is thought that this is because in certain people the T cells (see p. 96) fail to produce a chemical (lymphokine) which inhibits the fungus from germinating.

Recurrent candidiasis is difficult to treat. Recently a drug called ketokonazole, which is taken by mouth, has been used to treat candidal infections and also to treat recurrent infections. The treatment of recurrent infections is to give a small dose of ketokonazole each day for 6 months.

TRICHOMONIASIS

Trichomoniasis is the second of the sexually transmitted causes of vaginal inflammation. It is caused by a tiny parasite – *Trichomonas vaginalis* – which can only be seen through a microscope. It is about 20 micrometres in length (about the size of a pus cell), is globular in shape and has four moving threads at the front end, called flagellae, because of their whip-like action in propelling the organism. For this reason it is called a flagellate. Along its body from its headend, an undulating membrane stretches, which waves as the creature moves (Fig. 11/2).

The true incidence of trichomoniasis in a population is unknown,

Table 11/1 The treatment of candidiasis (medications in alphabetical order)

Proper (approved) name	*Trade (proprietary) names*	*Dosage*
CLOTRIMAZOLE		
Tablets	Canesten	Various regimens are recommended and all seem to be equally effective 1. 500mg tablet once, high in the vagina 2. two 100mg tablets at bedtime for 3 nights 3. one 100mg tablet at bedtime for 6 nights
Cream	Canesten Gyne-Lotrimin	One applicatorful high in the vagina each night for 6 nights
ECONAZOLE		
Tablets	Pevaryl	One 'ovule' placed high in the vagina at bedtime for 3 nights
Cream	Ecostatin	One applicatorful in the vagina at bedtime for 14 nights
KETOKONAZOLE		
Oral tablets	Nizoral	One tablet daily by mouth for 6 to 10 days
FLUCONAZOLE		
Oral tablets	Diflucan 150	One tablet (150mg) by mouth
MICONAZOLE		
Tablets	Gyno-Daktarin Monistat	One ovule high in the vagina at bedtime for 7 nights
Cream	Gyno-Daktarin	One applicatorful high in the vagina at bedtime for 7 nights
ISOCONAZOLE		
Tablets	Gyno-Travogen, Travogyn	One tablet high in the vagina
Cream	Gyno-Travogen, Travogyn	20g of cream high in the vagina
NYSTATIN		
Tablets	Mycostatin Nystan	One tablet high in the vagina night and morning for 14 days
Cream	Mycostatin Nilstat Nystan	One applicatorful high in the vagina night and morning for 14 days

If it is felt that the male is also infected, he should apply one of the creams to the glans of his penis each day for 10 days.

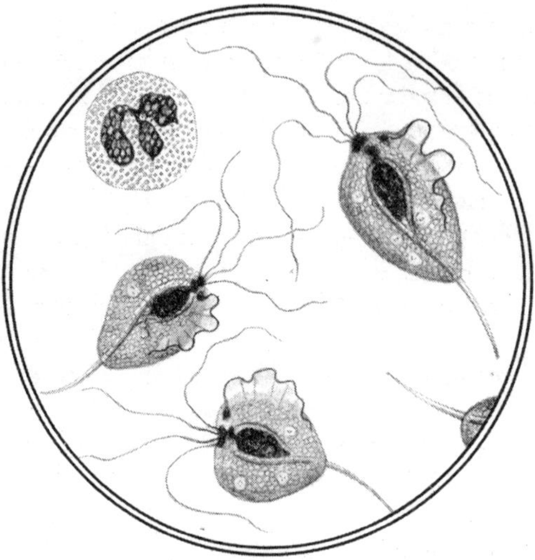

Fig. 11/2 Trichomonads seen through a microscope

but it has been estimated that it is present in the vaginas of between 5 and 20 per cent of sexually active women in the reproductive years of 15 to 49. By contrast, a survey of nearly 1000 virgins, aged 17 to 24, showed that only 2 per cent had trichomoniasis. This is the reason for including the disease among the sexually transmitted diseases. One calculation suggests that at any one time, over two million women in Britain have vaginal infestation with trichomoniasis, although most of these women have no symptoms and do not know that they are infected. Although the trichomonad usually inhabits the vagina, it occasionally enters the urethra and its associated extensions (which, you may remember, are called Skene's ducts), the bladder and Bartholin's glands.

Contrary to the popular belief that the vagina is a smooth-walled, well-lubricated tube, at least during sexual intercourse, it is, in fact, a most complex structure. Normally its two sides lie in touch with each other, and the wall itself is raised into complicated folds and clefts like a curtain of thick velvet. The importance of this concept is that the *Trichomonas vaginalis* organisms can lodge deep in the clefts where they obtain all the nourishment they want. In this warm, nutritious, protected environment they multiply.

There is increasing evidence that trichomoniasis is largely a sexually transmitted disease. As I mentioned, it is unusual to find it in virgins, and it is found more often in women who have had sexual intercourse. A typical story is for the woman to complain of a vaginal discharge, either white or greenish in colour, which smells 'fishy'. The discharge may be profuse in amount and is associated with discomfort or itching in the vagina. The symptoms begin 7 to 21 days after sexual intercourse. In some women, the itch is more severe than the discharge, the vaginal tenderness makes intercourse painful or impossible. In severe infections, the discharge is profuse and offensive. The vagina is intensely tender, and the vulva is reddened, swollen and inflamed, so that sexual intercourse is impossible, urination painful, walking uncomfortable and sitting a misery. Investigation of the discharge shows the presence of actively moving trichomonads, and smears taken from the male partner's urethra show where the infection came from.

In men, the urethra or its extensions may be infected, but in most cases the man has no symptoms. In some men, however, a urethritis occurs, and statistics suggest that about 10 to 20 per cent of cases of non-gonorrhoeal urethritis are due to infection by *Trichomonas vaginalis*. The importance of these observations is that when a woman is diagnosed as having trichomoniasis, both she and any sexual partners she may have should be treated, as between 30 and 70 per cent of the partners will also have the infection.

Trichomoniasis is said to be more frequent among prostitutes than puritans, blacks than whites, among pregnant than non-pregnant women, and among women in the developing nations. As well as this, investigations show that between 40 and 60 per cent of women with infectious gonorrhoea also harbour trichomonads in their vaginas. It is this additional infection that mainly accounts for the vaginal discharge these women complain about for, as was recorded earlier, the gonococcus cannot infect the vagina of an adult.

Although 10 to 20 per cent, or more, of women of reproductive age have trichomoniasis, in the majority the parasites live in harmony with the woman who unsuspectingly harbours them, and only cause symptoms from time to time. It is possible that frequent coitus may stimulate them, or that they cause symptoms only when the environment of the vagina changes for one reason or another.

Ten years ago, the development of a drug, metronidazole, revolutionized the treatment of trichomoniasis. The drug is effective when given by mouth, and no vaginal preparations are needed. But as it is specific for trichomoniasis, a diagnosis must be made before it is prescribed. This is done by taking a specimen of the discharge from inside the vagina. If the discharge is mixed with a drop of salt solution on a warmed slide, the parasite can be seen moving across the field, when looked at down a microscope. This method is useful if the parasite is seen, but its absence is not evidence that the patient has not got trichomoniasis. If any doubt exists, a specimen of the discharge is added to a test-tube containing a substance (Feinberg–Whittington medium) in which it grows excellently. This is incubated for 48 to 72 hours, when specimens of the solution are examined microscopically for trichomonads.

The treatment with metronidazole (Flagyl) is to give one tablet three times a day for 7 days, to the infected person and his, or her, partner. Recently a simpler treatment has become available. Four tablets of a drug called tinidazole (Fasigyn) are given in a single dose. This method seems as effective in treating trichomoniasis as the 7-day course. When taking either drug, alcohol should be avoided for the duration of the treatment and one day after because nausea, vomiting or abdominal cramps may occur.

A man is usually cured with a single course (or the 'one-shot' treatment) but trichomonads tend to persist in a woman because of the nature of her vagina. For this reason a woman can only be sure she is cured if further tests are made on swabs taken from her vagina just after her next menstrual period (and preferably after her next three menstrual periods) and these tests fail to show any trichomonads.

Fortunately, the cure rate is high. Over 90 per cent of infected women are cured with a single course of the drug, and the other 10 per cent are cured if a second treatment is given using a higher dose.

NON-SPECIFIC VAGINITIS (AMINE VAGINOSIS)

In this condition, the woman complains of a smelly, greyish coloured, irritant, vaginal discharge. Examination of a swab shows that neither candida nor trichomonas is present. The condition is believed to be due to the interaction of two kinds of bacteria which normally live in the vagina. The first is called *Gardnerella vaginalis* and the second are called anaerobes, as they do not need oxygen to grow. If the environment of the vagina is altered, an increased growth of both bacteria occurs, and a discharge results. As the anaerobes multiply they act on vaginal cells to release substances called amines, which are the cause of the 'fishy' smell of the discharge. The diagnosis of non-specific vaginitis (which is also called anaerobic vaginosis or amine vaginosis) can be made by the doctor in his surgery in most cases. The treatment is the same as that of trichomoniasis.

The extent to which non-specific vaginitis is a sexually transmitted disease is uncertain, but it seems that in a proportion of women, sexual contact is a factor.

Pubic lice

Pubic lice are relatives of head lice and may infect pubic hair. They are wingless insects the size of a pinhead, and are called crabs or crab-lice because of their appearance (Fig. 11/3a). Lice cannot jump and are transferred from person to person, usually during

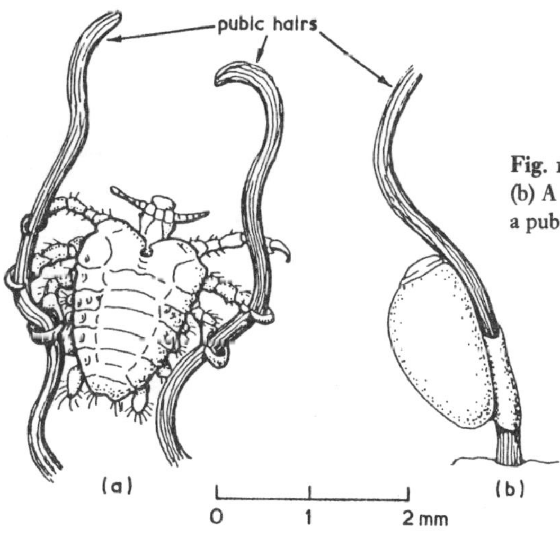

Fig. 11/3 (a) Pubic louse. (b) A louse egg (nit) on a pubic hair

sexual intercourse, when the pubic areas of both participants are in close contact. Occasionally they may be transferred from infested bedding or towels. The lice clasp pubic hair with claws on their hind feet, which makes them difficult to pick off. They feed by biting into the skin and sucking blood. This may cause itching and the infected person begins to scratch. The female louse lays about eight eggs each day and cements them to the hairs (Fig. 11/3b). After a week the nits hatch and the infestation spreads. Occasionally, head lice may also infect pubic hair.

Treatment of lice of any kind is to apply powders, shampoos or lotions containing 1 per cent gamma benzene hexachloride, or 0.5 per cent malathion, which is claimed to be less irritating to the skin.

Two methods of treatment are then recommended. In the first the pubic area is combed with a fine-tooth comb while the hair is still wet. This is rather time consuming but essential, and the infested person should stand on a large piece of newspaper which can be crumpled and burned, together with the nits. After combing, the pubic area should be rinsed thoroughly. This treatment should be repeated the following day.

The second method, which has been recommended by many experts, is to leave the lotion, cream or powder on the hairs for 24 hours, after which the person can have a shower or a bath. Usually one application is enough to kill the lice but if the infestation is heavy, the treatment is repeated in 7 days. Sexual partners should also be treated but there is no need to shave the person's pubic hair. If a pregnant woman has pubic lice gamma benzene should not be applied as it may be absorbed, stored in body fat and appear in the breast milk.

Molluscum contagiosum (Fig. 11/4)

Molluscum contagiosum is caused by a virus. The virus is transferred from person to person by close bodily contact, and enters the skin. In the skin it leads to a number of small, red, raised dimpled spots (papules) which contain a small amount of jelly-like material. Although molluscum contagiosum may occur anywhere on the body, the papules are most commonly found in the genital area. If the papules are unsightly or worry the person, they can be destroyed by pricking them with a sharp wooden stick dipped into phenol and squeezing out the jelly-like contents. Molluscum contagiosum has no serious consequences and is a very minor condition.

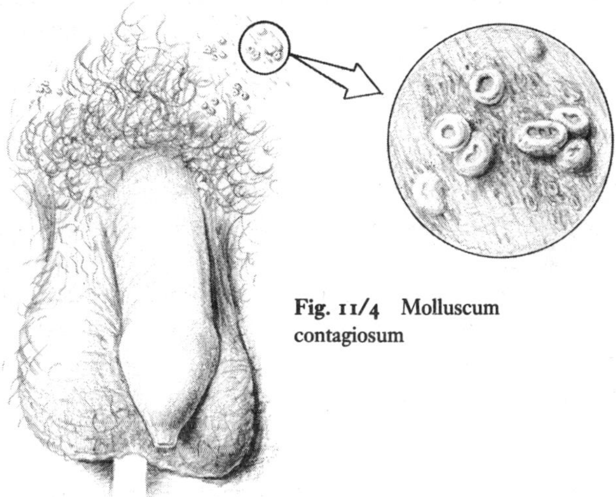

Fig. 11/4 Molluscum contagiosum

12. About the rare sexually transmitted diseases

Three sexually transmitted diseases are infrequently encountered in Western countries, but are more common in the developing, tropical countries. With increased travel, they may occur with greater frequency in Western nations in the future. The first of the diseases, called *chancroid*, is a legally notifiable 'venereal disease' in Britain and Australia, as well as some other countries. The other two diseases – *lymphogranuloma venereum*, which is caused by a sub-type of chlamydia, and *granuloma inguinale* – occur only rarely.

Chancroid

Chancroid is a sexually transmitted disease which usually occurs in the tropics and only rarely in temperate climates, but with increased air travel and movement of people, it is now being encountered in many countries.

It is an acute infectious disease of the genitals which is caused by a small organism called *Haemophilus ducreyi* after its discoverer, Dr Ducrey, who first identified it in an ulcer on a man's penis 90 years ago.

3 to 7 days after sexual intercourse with an infected partner, the man develops one or more small painful pimples on his penis, or the woman develops them on her labia. The pimples grow quickly, become very tender and then break down to form ulcers which have ragged edges and sloughing bases. They are soft, bleed easily and are very painful (you may remember that the primary lesion of syphilis, the chancre, is usually single, has a hard edge and is not painful). The lymph nodes in the groin become swollen and may become 'matted' together to form a large red painful swelling (Fig. 12/1).

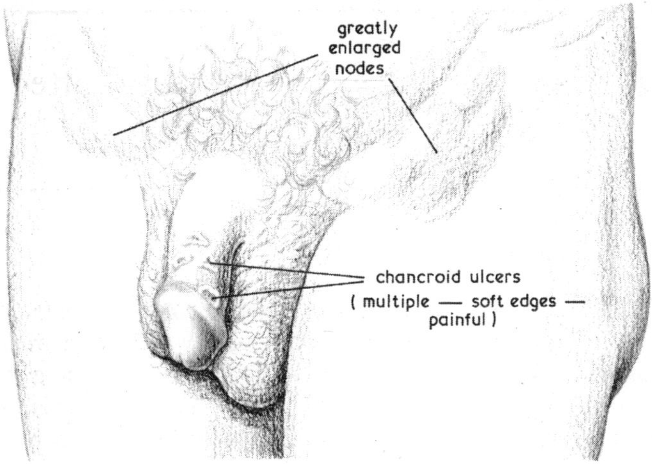

Fig. 12/1 Chancroid

The diagnosis is relatively easy, and is confirmed by taking a specimen from one of the ulcers and, after staining, looking down the microscope to find the organisms. In most cases this is unnecessary as the ulcers are fairly typical and the doctor gives treatment at once.

Treatment is to give sulphonamides, which are effective in curing chancroid, and have the advantage over the antibiotics that they do not suppress the early signs of syphilis.

An individual infected with chancroid may also be infected, at the same time, with syphilis, so that after curing the chancroid the patient must report any new lesion on his genitals, or any long-lasting skin rash (by this I mean a rash lasting for more than 14 days) and he should have routine blood tests made for syphilis at monthly intervals for 3 months.

Lymphogranuloma venereum (LGV)

LGV is caused by one of the family of chlamydia organisms which are also a cause of non-specific genital infection. Rarely encountered in Britain (only 32 cases were diagnosed in 1986), Canada or the USA (400 cases in 1986), it is more common in South East Asia and in Africa.

LGV is contracted by vaginal, oral or anal sexual contact with an infected person. Between 7 and 12 days (sometimes up to 12 weeks) the person develops a single blister on the penis, or on the external genitals of a woman. If the ulcer is on the penis or on the front part of a woman's genitals, the lymph nodes in the groin become enlarged, firm and rubbery, covered by shiny, bluish-red skin. The ulcers heal slowly with scarring, and the nodes either disappear or break down, releasing thick cheesy material through ragged holes in the skin.

The diagnosis is made by looking at the area and is confirmed by a test which demonstrates antibodies to chlamydia in the person's blood. Treatment is that of non-gonococcal urethritis (see p. 49) and if given before too much tissue has been damaged, results are good.

Granuloma inguinale

This is the least common sexually transmitted disease in the developed countries but is more common in East Asia, Latin America and sub-Saharan Africa. It is not very contagious and repeated sexual contact with an infected person does not always result in infection. Granuloma inguinale is caused by a bacterium called, until recently, *Donovania granulomatis*, after a Dr Donovan who described the condition. The infecting agent has now been given a new unpronounceable name!

If the infection occurs, some days, weeks or months later, small red lumps, or papules, appear on the genitals. These break down to form irregular ulcers, which can spread, if untreated, to affect most of the external genitals. The diagnosis is made by taking a swab from an ulcer, smearing it on a microscope slide and staining it. The treatment is that of the other rare sexually transmitted diseases.

13. A short history of the venereal diseases

Sexually transmitted diseases have probably existed for as long as humans have enjoyed sexual intercourse, but it must be admitted that the origins of the two sexually transmitted diseases which have been investigated for the longest period of time, namely gonorrhoea and syphilis, are obscure. According to an eminent venereologist of the nineteenth century, the Frenchman, Philippe Ricord, the first sentence of the Bible should have been 'In the beginning, God created the heavens, the earth, man and venereal diseases.'

Gonorrhoea, or a disease that was remarkably similar, is recorded in the Bible, where some of the earliest public health measures to prevent its spread are reported. About 3000 BC the Israelites, under Moses, made war on the Midianites, to avenge themselves for some real or imagined insult to them and to their God. In the first recorded account of a supernatural excuse being used to justify a war, the aim of which was to destroy the enemy's economic strength, the Israelites prospered, and won. As part of their victory they killed all the surviving male Midianites, and took the women and children captive, burning the Midianite villages and confiscating their herds of cattle and flocks of sheep. It was an utterly ruthless, vicious attack by one primitive tribe on another. They brought their booty, including the human booty, to a concentration camp on the plain of Moab near Jericho. It appears that the Israelites, flushed with victory, copulated with the Midianite women, for there was 'a plague amongst the congregation of the Lord'. Moses ordered that every Midianite woman 'that had known man by lying with him' should be killed, and every Israelite man who had copulated should be isolated 'outside the camp' for a period of 7 days. Interestingly, infection with gonorrhoea usually shows itself within 7 days of intercourse with an infected partner.

Oddly, gonorrhoea is not identifiable in Greek or Roman literature, nor does the medieval literature suggest any great concern. Perhaps the disease was so common that it was considered normal. Perhaps, as disease at that time was considered to be due to an act of God because of man's sin, it may have been thought not worth recording. In England by the twelfth century, there was some concern about the disease, and London brothel-keepers were forbidden to supply clients with women who suffered from 'the perilous infirmity of burning'. The term burning was an abbreviation of the Norman–French name for gonorrhoea, 'hot-piss' or 'la chaude pisse'. The current popular name for gonorrhoea – the clap – only became fashionable about two centuries later, by which time, with a relaxation of sexual morality, the disease had become widespread.

By this time syphilis had appeared in Europe to complicate the picture, and for the next 300 years, until 1793, gonorrhoea and syphilis were considered to be manifestations of a single 'venereal' disease. In part this confusion was increased by the well-known and respected physician, John Hunter, who in 1767 'proved' that the two conditions were one. Hunter believed that the clinical appearance of the disease depended on where the poison was inoculated. If it entered the urethra the victim developed gonorrhoea; if it infected the penis, the victim developed a syphilitic ulcer. To prove his point he took some pus from a patient who had gonorrhoea and placed it in his urethra. Within 7 days he had developed gonorrhoea, and within a month he had developed the skin rash of syphilis. The proof was there – syphilis and gonorrhoea were the same disease.

It was of course, no proof at all, for the pus had contained the germs that cause gonorrhoea, *Neisseria gonorrhoeae*, and those that cause syphilis, *Treponema pallidum*. Unfortunately, Hunter was so eminent, and his views so respected, that his findings were accepted and further progress was delayed until 1793, when Benjamin Bell in Edinburgh identified that there were two diseases. Unfortunately for John Hunter the syphilis he had acquired led to illness in his last years and eventually to his death. Benjamin Bell was more cautious. He inoculated medical students, and proved that there were two separate sexually transmitted diseases – gonorrhoea and syphilis.

William Wallace, in Dublin about 15 years later, carried the identification one step farther. He proved that the skin rash of syphilis, as well as the initial infection, an ulcer on the penis, was highly infectious. He did this by inoculating patients in the free wards of the hospital in which he worked. So much for the ethics of medical practice at the time! Wallace had one other claim to fame. This is in the treatment of syphilis. At that time the only remedy, which was largely ineffectual, was to give mercury, either rubbed into the skin or taken by mouth, in the form of 'blue pills'. Mercury, of course, is very toxic, as the experience of fish eaters in Minamata Bay in Japan has shown recently. Mercury given to cure syphilis caused teeth to fall out, kidney damage and mental decay – all of which were attributed to the progress of the disease, not to the treatment. Wallace argued that the salt of another element might be even more successful. He chose to give potassium iodide, which led to the medical students' rhyme:

If you lose your faith in God
Put your trust in pot. iod!

Unfortunately, the use of potassium iodide in the treatment of syphilis was only marginally better, if at all better, than the use of mercury.

Syphilis is one of a group of diseases called treponematoses, because the organisms that cause them are tiny corkscrew-shaped germs calls treponemes. In tropical areas a common treponematosis is yaws. Yaws is spread by bodily – not sexual – contact, in conditions of poor hygiene and infrequent washing. The disease is chronic and large ulcers form over the body. It usually only affects small children and persists for years if it is not treated. In tropical America, another variety of treponematosis, called pinta, develops in primitive people in rural areas. In this disease young persons aged 10 to 25, rather than young children, are affected. Once again the disease is spread by body contact, by rubbing against an infected lesion, and not by sexual intercourse.

Syphilis is the only treponematosis that is spread by sexual intercourse. It is also the only one of the diseases that is a potential killer, but because of the existence of other treponemal diseases its origin is obscure.

Until some 5 years after the return of Columbus from America, syphilis was unknown in Europe; but after that time, for two centuries, the disease raged as an epidemic throughout the continent. Those who believe that syphilis was brought back to Europe by Columbus's sailors, claim that America was given to Europe so that the Europeans might plunder it, and later settle their excess population in its empty lands, and in return America gave Europe a particularly damaging disease. This new disease spread to all parts of the world from its introduction into Barcelona by sailors infected by the Indians of the Isle of Española in the Caribbean.

The first description of the disease was by a Portuguese physician, Ruy Diaz de Isla, who worked in Barcelona. He was called to treat some of Columbus's men who were covered with a pustular skin rash and had snail-track, or serpentine, ulcers on their mouths and throats. He first termed the disease 'Indian measles' because the skin rash resembled measles, but was not exactly like it. Later he called it the 'serpentine disease'. He described it as 'a disease, previously unknown, unseen and undescribed, which first appeared in the city and spread thence throughout the world'. About 15 years after Diaz saw the first cases, the disease was widespread in all European nations, and he wrote a book which he called *A Treatise on the Serpentine Malady*. In this book he wrote:

> It has pleased divine justice to give and send down upon us unknown afflictions, never seen nor recognized nor found in medical books, such as this serpentine disease . . . at the time that the Admiral don Xristoual Colon [Columbus] arrived in Spain, the Catholic sovereigns were in the city of Barcelona. And when they went to give them an account of their voyage and of what they had discovered, immediately the city began to be infected and the aforesaid disease spread as was seen later on through long experience.

The alternative view of the origin of syphilis is that the treponeme group of diseases existed in Europe (as they did in Africa and America) but were so mild that they were unrecognized. Then in the last decade of the fifteenth century they suddenly became virulent and sexually transmissible. Whatever the origin, after 1494 syphilis rapidly spread throughout Europe. In the autumn of 1494, Charles VIII of France invaded Italy to seize the throne of Naples. His army consisted of mercenaries, including Spanish mercenaries, and they laid siege to Naples. Accompanying the army, as was the custom, went a collection of female camp followers, known as 'bagages' (Fig. 13/1). The king of Naples had also obtained mercenary soldiers to defend his city and these included a number of Spanish soldiers. There was little fighting but much fornication by both armies, and by the spring of 1495 a new plague had affected both the defenders and the attackers. The plague was the serpentine disease of Diaz. The new disease was so severe and so many of his troops were affected, that Charles was forced to abandon his siege and retreat from Italy. With his army he took the new unnamed disease.

As the mercenaries returned to their homelands they fornicated on the way, and those they infected spread the new disease. It passed down from man to woman and then to another man and another woman with great rapidity. Sexually transmissible, the new disease was transmitted by frequent fornication with different partners. As

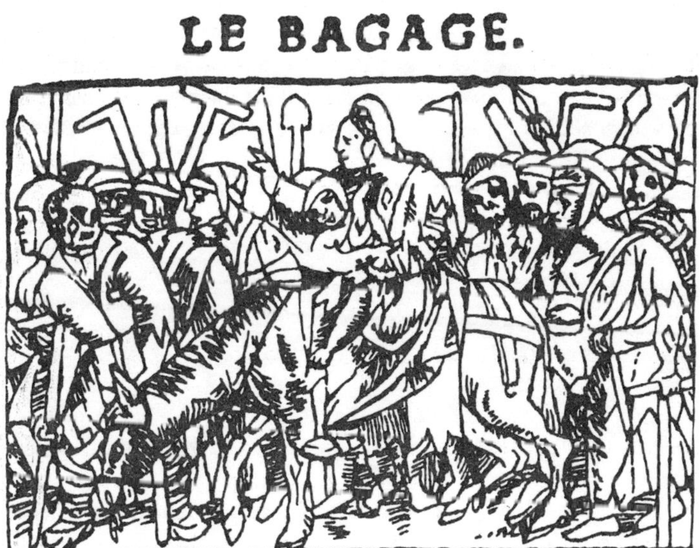

Fig. 13/1 Le Bagage, or the camp follower. 'The impedimenta of the Army. Triumph of the high and mighty, Dame Syphilis, Queen of the Fountain of Love' (Lyons, 1539), from W. A. Pusey, *The History and Epidemiology of Syphilis*, 1933 (Courtesy of Charles C. Thomas, Springfield, Illinois)

the people of each country became infected, each tried to put the blame for the new and terrifying disease on its neighbour. The Italians called it the Spanish disease. The French, who were first infected in 1495, called it the Italian or Neapolitan disease.

By 1496 the disease was infecting large numbers of people in Germany, France and Switzerland. It reached Holland and Greece in 1496, and England in 1497, where it was called the French disease. In the same year Perkin Warbeck, who claimed to be the Duke of York, had invaded the north of England from Scotland, with 1400 disreputable followers, and with the support of James IV of Scotland. Among these mercenaries were some from Charles's army. The invasion was a failure and the motley regiment was driven back into Scotland. They took with them the new serpentine disease. In Aberdeen the disease took hold so rapidly that by 1498 the town's leaders became dismayed. Recognizing that the disease was spread by sexual intercourse, they published a regulation in which they ordered 'all light women to desist from their vice and sin of venery' on pain of being branded. The regulation was ineffective. Sex continued rampant and by 1507 the authorities of Aberdeen ordered that 'diligent inquisitions be taken of all infected persons with this strange sickness of Napolis for the safety of the town'. The infected were ordered 'to keep quiet in their houses'!

By 1500 the disease had spread to Hungary and Russia, and was being taken to India by the Portuguese explorers under Vasco de Gama. It reached China in 1505 and Japan a year later where it was called 'manka bassam' or the Portuguese disease.

The epidemic raged like a bush fire. Because of the virulence of the organisms, or the lack of resistance by the people to the new disease, it was viciously severe. The primary lesion was hardly noticed when compared with the secondary lesions, which developed 6 to 8 weeks later. These caused severe illnesses, and often deaths, as the pustular ulcerated skin rashes, and the snail track lesions in the mouth, the throat and the genitals spread unabated. Such evidence as there is suggests that many thousands died. As well as causing death, the skin lesions were highly infectious and even non-sexual contact with an infected person caused the infection to spread. Such was the concern of the people that the Holy Church was petrified, and a patron saint was appointed to whom victims might pray. By a coincidence he was also the patron saint of France and Paris. It seemed that the French were to be blamed for the disease, which in a way was logical, for it was the French king's mercenary army which had started its rapid spread. St Denis, patron saint of Paris and France, became the patron saint of the new disease and in a book published between 1496 and 1500, he is seen standing by and interceding with the Virgin on behalf of pock-marked sufferers from the new plague (Fig. 13/2).

Treatment seemed ineffective, although mercury was used in the hope that it would help. Prayer also seemed ineffective. The disease continued to spread with increasing severity. In the early years severe ulcerating, pustular rashes on the skin and in the mouth predominated. They were associated with fevers and aching pains deep in the bones. As time passed, the rash became less obvious, but many victims infected earlier developed gummy ulcerated swellings in their bones, which often ate away the cartilage of the palate and nose. By now, too, mercury toxicity was causing baldness and loss of teeth. Bone pains, which were gnawing and occured at night, persisted, keeping the victim awake and screaming.

It took over a hundred years for the severity of the disease to moderate, and the pattern seen today to evolve. But during that century, the disease rampaged and together with bubonic plague and enteric fevers laid waste many families.

The name syphilis was first given to the disease in 1530, when Dr Fracastor, a physician and poet of Verona in Italy, wrote a poem about a young swineheard, called Syphilis, who angered the god Apollo, by building forbidden altars on a sacred hill. As a punishment Apollo inflicted a terrible disease on him, in which ulcers of the skin, or buboes, were the main feature. Fracastor wrote:

> He first wore buboes dreadful to the sight
> First felt strange pains, and sleepless passed the night
> From him the malady received its name
> The neighbouring shepherds catch'd the spreading flame.

The title page of Fracastor's poem reads 'Syphilis sive Morbus Gallicus'. This is translated as 'Syphilis or the French disease'. There can be no doubt that Dr Fracastor had seen several cases of 'serpentine disease', and he wrote his poem to give it a proper name.

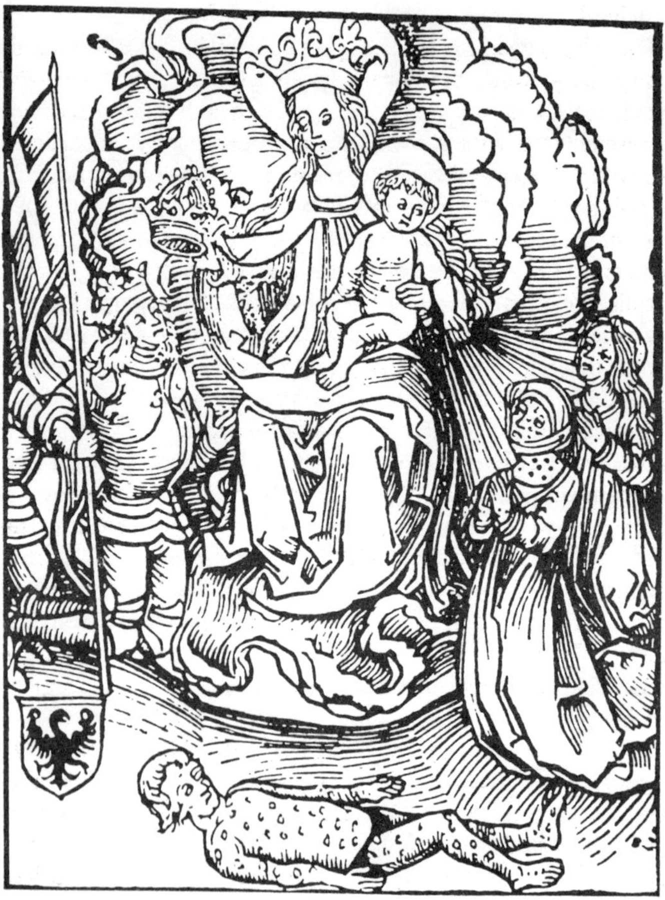

Fig. 13/2 St Denis supplicates the Virgin Mary to help a victim of the new disease, (Originally in Grunpeck's book published between 1496 and 1500.) from W. A. Pusey, *The History and Epidemiology of Syphilis*, 1933 (Courtesy of Charles C. Thomas, Springfield, Illinois)

As the Italians claimed the disease had been introduced by the French (whom they detested) it seemed a good idea to Fracastor to give the disease a second name, the French disease. His poem was widely read and the disease generally acquired the name, Syphilis, which had none of the pejorative connotations of the earlier name. It has been called syphilis ever since, a sad tribute to a sacrilegious swineherd.

The alternative name, the great-pox, which was chosen to distinguish it from the other epidemic – the small-pox – was introduced in England some time in the sixteenth century because of the resemblance in the two diseases, of skin lesions which pocked the skin with sores and ulcers. But because the painful symptoms and the number of deaths from syphilis were so much more severe than those of small-pox, it was given the name of the great-pox. By the eighteenth century, the great-pox had become the common term for syphilis. It had, in general, been shortened to 'the pox' which is what it is called today. A student's song about 'The Good Ship Venus' records that one of the sailors 'caught the syph. at Tenerife, the pox in the Canaries'. He was clearly a lusty sailor.

Throughout its recorded history, the main cause of the spread of the disease has been casual fornication, usually with prostitutes. Consequently, travellers, soldiers and sailors have been particularly at risk, as were the rakes and dandies of eighteenth-century England, whose promiscuity was neither in doubt nor unheralded. However, syphilis can affect a bishop or a 'baggage' and neither kings nor the rulers of the earth have been spared. There is good evidence that Henry VIII's inability to have a healthy child and the mental disturbances of his later years were due to syphilis acquired in his youth.

By the nineteenth century, a revulsion from the overt sexuality of the two earlier centuries had made venereal disease one of the unmentionable matters, in Britain at least, together with women's legs and breasts. This in no way reduced the incidence or spread of the sexually transmitted disease, which in a man was considered indiscreet or perhaps degrading, but in a woman was treated as a crime. The double standard towards sexuality, which regrettably persists today, received a majestic reinforcement from mid-Victorian paternalistic, authoritarian 'morality'.

Despite the widespread prevalence of syphilis, no documentation was made of its frequency, except among soldiers. In the mid-nineteenth century, rates of 70 to 120 per 1000 men were reported from the armies of the USA, Britain, Prussia and France. By the onset of the First World War, the rates had decreased by 20 to 45 per cent, as the conspiracy of secrecy and the punitive attitude of authority towards infected men diminished. During this period, too, education was becoming more widespread, particularly of the working classes, who are recorded as having two or three times the chances of contracting the disease, although this statistic may be artificial as many wealthier syphilitics were treated by private doctors, and the disease was not reported to the public health authorities.

The available evidence suggests that the decline in the number of new cases of syphilis and gonorrhoea reported each year between 1850 and 1910 was real, and was related more to social factors than to control of the disease, which was rudimentary, or to treatment, which was ineffectual.

In 1910, for the first time, a treatment was devised that had the possibility of curing syphilis. This was Ehrlich's 'magic bullet', or salvarsan. Salvarsan, which was an arsenical and given by injection, seemed to offer a cure. At the same time the development of microscopy had enabled doctors to diagnose the disease early, and a blood test had been devised by Wassermann to detect those in whom the clinical signs of syphilis had disappeared, but who still had the disease. It appeared that a new, and more scientific period in the management of syphilis was about to begin.

It has not worked out that way, at all. In fact in the last decade, in all Western nations, there has been an upsurge in the incidence of syphilis. In the USA for example, infectious syphilis is now more common than poliomyclitis, tuberculosis and the other infectious diseases which, not so long ago, were considered a threat to mankind.

It is difficult to determine exactly how common the sexually transmitted diseases are, as a large number of infected people are treated by private doctors who feel they have neither the duty to report, nor do they have the wish to embarrass a paying patient by reporting the disease to the public health authorities. Yet if this new epidemic is to be controlled, the names of all infected persons must be notified, so that their sexual partner or partners can be contacted, before they in turn infect other people. The purpose of notifying the public health authorities is not to embarrass or to punish the individual, but to prevent the disease from spreading. It is a public health matter, not a moral matter.

The most accurate study of the prevalence of syphilis in the population of a nation was made by testing the blood of all men aged 18 to 35 who were drafted into the USA armed forces in the Second World War. From these data, it was estimated by Drs Parran and Vonderleht that 24 people in every 1000 alive in the United States in 1942 had syphilis, although in most the disease had been treated and was non-infectious.

In most Western nations from which accurate data are available, the highest number of new cases of syphilis occurred during the war years, reaching a peak in 1945–6 just after demobilization. A dramatic fall occurred between 1946 and 1950 and the lower incidence has been maintained since that date, but fluctuations have occurred. For example, in the USA the number of cases per 100 000 of the population doubled from 5 per 100 000 in the late 1950s to 10 per 100 000 during the Vietnam War years and has remained at about this level. Since 1950, in Britain, the number of cases of syphilis reported has varied between 1 and 2 per 100 000 of the population, a relatively low level (Fig. 13/3). In Sweden the number of cases per 100 000 of the population was 1 per 100 000 in the late 1950s. It rose to a peak of 6 per 100 000 in the mid-1960s and has subsequently fallen to 5 per 100 000 inhabitants.

The decline of reported syphilis observed in the developed nations has not been observed in the developing nations, where syphilis seems to be increasing in incidence. In fact the world total of persons infected with syphilis is astonishingly high. A committee of UNESCO estimated that in 1969 there were between 20 and 50 million cases of venereal syphilis in the world. This is probably an underestimate because of under-reporting, and the number has increased since that date.

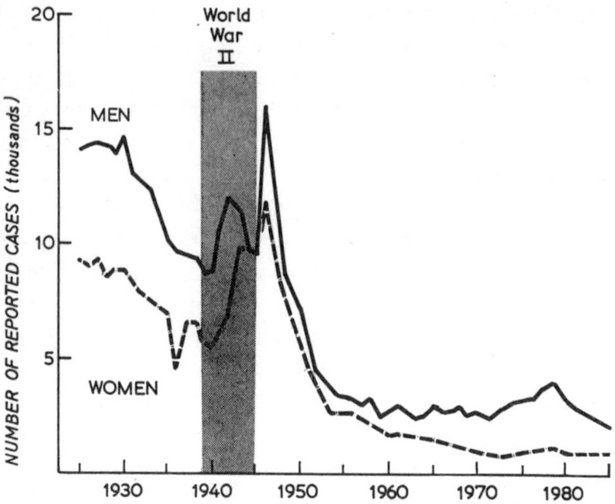

Fig. 13/3 The decline in the incidence of syphilis in England and Wales since 1946

Gonorrhoea

The present situation with regard to gonorrhoea is more disturbing. The World Health Organization calculates that 10 cases of gonorrhoea occur for every case of syphilis, which means that currently there may be between 200 million and 500 million cases annually. The disease has reached world-wide epidemic proportions. As with syphilis, official figures must be treated with reserve, for in most nations, patients with gonorrhoea seek treatment from private physicians and the disease is not reported.

The integrity of private doctors in reporting gonorrhoea varies from country to country. A survey carried out in the USA in 1966 by Dr MacKenzie-Pollock, for example, showed that 80 per cent of cases of gonorrhoea were treated by private doctors, but only one case in nine was reported to the health authorities. More recent information indicates that little change has occurred. Because of the failure of many doctors to notify cases of gonorrhoea, the published figures, which relate to 'public clinics', do not give the true incidence of the disease. Yet in several Western countries an increase in cases of gonorrhoea has been reported. Perhaps the most spectacular rise

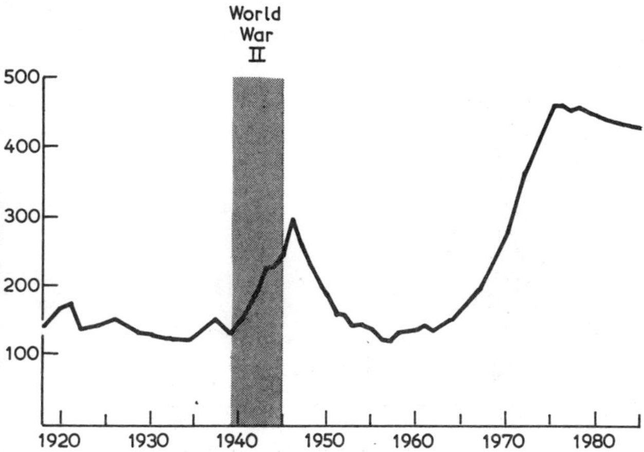

Fig. 13/4 Reported cases of gonorrhoea (probably about one-tenth of people infected) per 100 000 population in the USA 1919–85 (WHO data)

has been in the USA where the number of cases reported each year rose from 150 per 100 000 in 1960 to 430 per 100 000 in 1978 (Fig. 13/4). This equates to over 1 million *reported* cases in 1975 and, as has been mentioned, fewer than half of the cases are reported. In England and Wales a small increase occurred between 1960 and 1978 but since then fewer cases are being diagnosed (Fig. 13/5).

In Sweden, perhaps because of more frequent reporting by doctors, the rate rose from 250 per 100 000 inhabitants in 1960 to 500 per 100 000 in 1970. Since 1970 a considerable fall has occurred and in 1980 the rate was 250 per 100 000. It is believed that the fall in reported cases of gonorrhoea in Sweden since 1970 is due to the recognition by the public of the fact that over half of women infected with gonorrhoea have no symptoms. They constitute a 'hidden reservoir'. In Sweden, because of a much more open attitude to sexually transmitted diseases, and a reduction in the 'shame' of having caught one, infected men are more able to talk with their sexual partners and advise them to be examined. The women feel less inhibited about going for an examination. This has

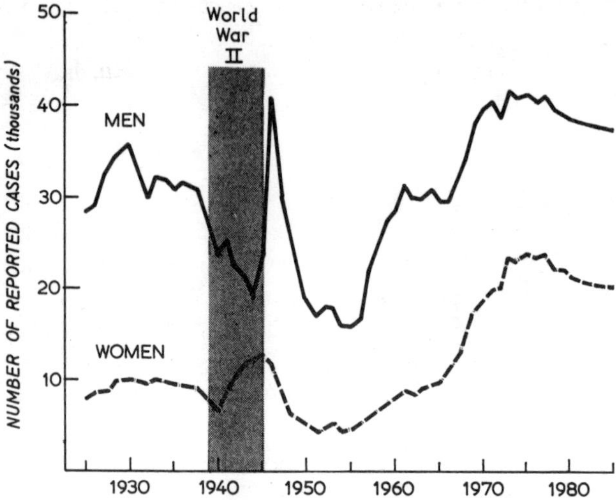

Fig. 13/5 The incidence of new cases of gonorrhoea in England and Wales since 1925 as reported from sexually transmitted diseases clinics

reduced the 'reservoir' of symptomless, infected women and the number of cases of gonorrhoea is declining.

Against the trend of an increasing number of cases of gonorrhoea occurring each year among men and women in many Western nations, reports from China, Eastern Europe and the USSR suggest that fewer cases of gonorrhoea are being reported.

In all nations reporting statistics of sexually transmitted diseases, increasing numbers of young adults are being infected with gonorrhoea and NGGI, and recent surveys in Western nations show that over 66 per cent of all cases occur in people under the age of 25. Among this age-group between three and five times as many men as women are infected. This higher incidence among men may be partly spurious, because of the lack of symptoms in some infected women.

The rise in incidence of gonorrhoea in the past 10 years among young people is due to their increased sexual activity. In all Western countries more young people are becoming sexually active at an earlier age. Studies made in the mid-1980s in Britain, Scandinavia and the USA show that by age 16, 20 per cent of young men and 13 per cent of young women have been sexually active. By the age of 19 the proportion of sexually active men has risen to 85 per cent and that of women to 55 per cent. Many people may deplore this, but the facts are that it is occurring and, unless there is a sudden, dramatic change in sexual attitudes, it is likely to persist.

Non-gonococcal genital infection (NGGI)

This sexually transmitted disease has been known to infect men from the time that gonorrhoea could be diagnosed by looking at a swab taken from the pus from his urethra. When the pus was examined from a number of men who had the symptoms of gonorrhoea, no gonococci were found. This led to the discovery of a new disease, which was called non-gonococcal urethritis or NGU.

It is only in the past 20 years that it has become clear that NGU is often caused by a small organism called chlamydia. This organism infects women too, but the woman's urethra is usually not infected; instead the cells lining the canal in her cervix are infected. Lurking in these cells, chlamydia causes no symptoms, but it may infect a man with whom she has sexual intercourse. The disease is now called NGGI.

More seriously for the woman's health, the infection may spread upwards through the uterus to infect the Fallopian tubes, so damaging them that pregnancy becomes impossible.

NGGI is now 3–5 times as common as gonorrhoea, in the developed countries of the world.

HIV infection

The human immunodeficiency virus, which causes AIDS, was first reported in the USA in 1981. Originating in Central Africa, where it was mainly spread through prostitutes, it reached the Caribbean and infected homosexual men, who brought it to the USA and from there it has spread to most other developed countries. Since 1981, HIV infection has spread amongst the at-risk populations very rapidly. In the Western world, these groups are homosexual and bisexual men (75 per cent); intravenous drug users (20 per cent), and more recently women. In Central Africa, men and women are affected in equal proportions.

In its short history, HIV has infected upwards of 8.5 million people. What will happen in the future is unknown but there is early evidence that the infection rate is falling. Whether this is due to more people adopting safer sexual practices, or to changes in the virulence of the virus is unknown. In spite of intense research there is, as yet, no cure. The available drugs improve the quality of life and may delay death, but they do not eliminate the virus.

What is different about the AIDS pandemic, from earlier sexually transmitted disease epidemics, like syphilis, is that today there are powerful microbiological techniques which, with great speed, have identified the virus, and established factors that increase its virulence.

Reducing the effect of the STDs

Rather than uttering plaintive, platitudinous prophesies about moral decay, the moralists should be bending their energies to reducing the effects of the greater sexuality of young people. These effects include the spread of sexually transmissible diseases and an increase in extra-marital, unwanted pregnancies. Both could be reduced by better education about human sexuality and about sexually transmitted diseases, by removing the stigma of seeking medical help if a young person catches gonorrhoea, NGGI or syphilis, so that he or she seeks medical aid at once, without fear of shame. This demands that moralists treat the sexually transmissible diseases as infectious diseases, like every other infectious disease.

Medically, sexually transmitted diseases should be managed in the same way as measles, poliomyelitis or food poisoning. The second effect of increased sexuality, that of unwanted pregnancy, could be reduced by better education and by better distribution of contraceptives, which should be freely available. If condoms were freely available to all adolescents and it was the fashion to use one when having casual coitus, the incidence of NGGI and gonorrhoea would decline. Today in the English-speaking nations, these two diseases are more likely to be contracted by fornicating with an acquaintance or a friend than by copulating with a prostitute.

A survey in the USA showed that 20 per cent of prostitutes had gonorrhoea and 2 per cent had infectious syphilis. In the nations of

Europe, where prostitution is under stricter control and brothels are usual, the infection rate among professional prostitutes is said to be lower.

Unless the medical control is scrupulous, it is unlikely to reduce the transmission of the diseases. Strict medical control means that vaginal, cervical, urethral and throat swabs are taken each week from each prostitute, and rectal swabs are also taken if the woman offers anal intercourse. Women found to have gonorrhoea or NGGI are treated and must not work during treatment. As some clients of prostitutes (or boyfriend or husband) may be symptomless carriers of gonorrhoea or NGGI, new infections may occur in the interval between screening, and the woman may infect other men. The best control will be obtained if brothels are registered and must conform to a routine of weekly medical checks and if clients wear condoms. However, street-walkers, who usually refuse or do not seek medical checks, are likely to continue to infect numbers of men.

Homosexual men appear to be an increasing source of new cases, both of syphilis and gonorrhoea. Whether the increase is real or apparent is not certain. In Britain this is because alterations in the law in 1967, which made homosexuality between consenting adult males no longer a crime, made it possible for homosexuals to seek treatment without fear of prosecution; but it may also be a real increase. Since between 5 and 10 per cent of all males are homosexual or bisexual and since as many homosexuals are as sexually promiscuous as are heterosexuals, it is not unexpected that cases of sexually transmitted diseases will occur in the homosexual community. It is not known whether homosexual promiscuity is due to childhood emotional disturbances which prevent the man from forming any lasting relationship with another person, or whether the contempt shown by society and the penalties it imposes on known homosexuals, are the major factors in homosexual promiscuity. Research in this area is urgently needed.

Further reading

The following relate to comments and discussions within the content of the book and are listed by Chapter number.

Chapter 2

STATISTICAL DATA

Clinical returns for new cases by diagnosis are published each year in Britain in the *British Medical Journal* and the *British Journal of Venereal Diseases*. In the USA the morbidity and mortality weekly reports published in the *Journal of the American Medical Association* provide information.

CHANGES IN SEXUAL BEHAVIOUR

Brandt, E. N. (1982). Physicians and sexually transmitted disease: a call to action. *Journal of the American Medical Association*, **248**, 2032–3.

Catterall, R. D. (1981). Biological effects of sexual freedom. *Lancet*, **ii**, 315–19.

Farrell, C. (1978). *My Mother Said.* Routledge and Kegan Paul, London.

Henderson, R. H. (1975). Venereal disease. A national health problem. *Clinical Obstetrics and Gynecology*, **18**, 223–53.

Jaffe, F. S. (1976). *International Family Planning*, **2**, 3–7.

Kantner, J. F. and Zelnik, M. (1972). *Family Planning Perspectives*, **4**, 5–8.

Kantner, J. F. and Zelnik, M. (1977). *Family Planning Perspectives*, **9**, 55–9.

Knightley, P. (1984). The *Sunday Times* report on Sex, Love and Marriage 1984, in association with Dr W. James and MORI. *Sunday Times*, 29 April.

Schofield, M. (1975). *Sexual Behaviour of Young People.* Allen Lane, London.

Chapter 3

Further detailed descriptions of the female and male genital tract anatomy may be obtained from the following titles by Derek Llewellyn-Jones:

Fundamentals of Obstetrics and Gynaecology, Volume 2, 5th edition, 1990.

Everywoman, 5th edition, 1989. (Both titles are published by Faber and Faber, London.)

Every Man, 1986 (Published by Oxford University Press, Oxford.)

Chapter 4

Dunlop, E. M. C. (1983). Chlamydia genital infection and its complications. *British Journal of Hospital Medicine*, 6–11.

Editorial (1974). Promiscuity and infertility. *British Medical Journal*, **ii**, 501–2.

Editorial (1981). Non-specific genital infection. *British Medical Journal*, **ii**, 161.

Felman, Y. M. and Nikitas, J. A. (1981). Non-gonococcal urethritis – a review. *Journal of the American Medical Association*, **245**, 381–6.

Schachter, J. and Grossman, M. (1981). Chlamydia infections. *Annual Review Medicine*, **32**, 45–64.

Chapter 5

Donovan, B. (1984). Gonorrhoea in a Sydney house of prostitution. *Medical Journal of Australia*, **i**, 268–71.

Chapter 6

GENITAL WARTS

Adler, M. W. (1984). *British Medical Journal*, **i**, 213–16.

Beutner, K. R., *et al.* (1989). Patient applied Podofilox for the treatment of genital warts. *Lancet*, **i**, 831–4

Chapter 7

Editorial (1983). Herpes – hype or hope? *British Medical Journal*, **i**, 1767–8

Kilbrick, S. (1980). Herpes simplex infection at term. *Journal of the American Medical Association*, **243**, 157–60.

Oakes, J. K. (1983). *Herpes – The Facts*. Penguin Books, Harmondsworth. (This is an excellent clear and unemotional account of herpes, written in lucid English.)

Votrer, L. A., *et al.* (1982). Recurrent genital herpes in pregnancy. *American Journal of Obstetrics and Gynecology*, **143**, 75–84.

Chapter 8

RISK OF INFECTION

Schrober, R., *et al.* (1983). How infectious is syphilis? *British Journal of Venereal Disease*, **59**, 217–19.

NORWEGIAN STUDY

Gjestland, T. (1955). *Acta Dermato-Venereologica (Stockholm)*, **35**, Supp 34.

CONGENITAL AND PRENATAL SYPHILIS

Charles, D. (1983). Syphilis. *Clinics in Obstetrics and Gynaecology*, **26**, 125–37.

Chapter 9

AIDS

Adler, M. and Weller, I. V. D. (1984). AIDS – sense not fear. *British Medical Journal*, i, 1177–8.

Beverley, P. and Sattentau, Q. (1987) Immunology of AIDS. *British Medical Journal*, **294**, 1536–9.

Centres for Disease Control (1982). AIDS – precautions for clinical and laboratory staff. *MMWR* 31/577–580.

Editorial (1983). AIDS – two years later. *New England Journal of Medicine*, **309**, 609–10.

Madeley, T. (1987) Having AIDS. *British Medical Journal*, **295**, 320–2.

Steel, M. (1988). Report 4th International AIDS Conference, 1988. *Lancet*, **ii**, 54–5.

Timbs, O. and Fraser, L. (1984). On the trace of the cause and cure of AIDS. *The Times*, 6 April.

Chapter 10

VIRAL HEPATITIS

Tedder, R. S. (1983). Viral hepatitis as a sexually transmitted disease. *British Journal of Hospital Medicine*, 1, 23–5.

Chapter 11

VAGINITIS

Dawson, S. G. and Harries, J. R. W. (1983). Gardnerella vaginalis and non-specific vaginitis. *British Journal of Hospital Medicine*, 1, 28–37.
Eschenbach, D. (1983). Vaginal infection. *Clinics in Obstetrics and Gynaecology*, **26**, 186–202.
Llewellyn-Jones, D. (1990). *Fundamentals of Obstetrics and Gynaecology*, 5th edn., Volume 2, Gynaecology (Chapter 15). Faber and Faber, London.
Sobel, J. (1986) Candida infections. *New England Journal of Medicine*, **315**, 1455–5.

Index